All
God's
Mistakes

Charles L. Bosk

ALL GOD'S MISTAKES

GENETIC COUNSELING IN A PEDIATRIC HOSPITAL

The University of Chicago Press
Chicago and London

The University of Chicago Press, Chicago 60637
The University of Chicago Press, Ltd., London
© 1992 by The University of Chicago
All rights reserved. Published 1992
Paperback edition 1995
Printed in the United States of America

01 00 99 98 97 96 95   2 3 4 5 6

ISBN (cloth): 0-226-06681-9
ISBN (paper): 0-226-06682-7

Library of Congress Cataloging-in-Publication Data

Bosk, Charles L.
    All God's mistakes : genetic counseling in a pediatric hospital /
Charles L. Bosk.
        p.   cm.
    Includes bibliographical references and index.
    1. Genetic counseling.   2. Genetic counselors.   I. Title.
    [DNLM: 1. Ethics, Medical—United States.   2. Genetic Counseling—
    United States. QZ 50 B743a]
    RB155.7.B67   1992
    616'.042—dc20
    DNLM/DLC
    for Library of Congress   91-36938
                                                                        CIP

In memory of my Uncle Joseph Bosk, a man with vast
intellectual interests, but few words.
I miss them all.

CONTENTS

ix
Contents

ACKNOWLEDGMENTS

My first debt is to the workers in and the families who used the genetic counseling services of Nightingale Children's Center. Without their cooperation, this work could never have been done. I am deeply grateful that under difficult circumstances I was allowed to observe so many medical encounters in which privacy was the original expectation. The conventions of confidentiality and anonymity which govern field research prevent a more extensive thanks, but my gratitude runs deeper than these few spare words indicate.

The fieldwork was sponsored by a grant from the United States Public Health Services, National Institute of Child Health and Development, as well as by the Picker Program for Humane Qualities in Medicine.

A book that takes as long to complete as this one did perforce involves the help of many others. At the University of Pennsylvania, I have been blessed with helpful colleagues. Harold Bershady, Renée Fox, and Seth Kreimer read multiple drafts with a gentle but critical eye. At early stages of this work, Alex Capron provided encouragement and guidance. An informal seminar on work with Ivar Berg, Fred Block, Richard Ingersoll, Jerry Jacobs, Robin Leidner, Werner Van Der Ohe, Victoria Smith, and Rosemary Wright convinced me to highlight the work of Everett Hughes in this volume.

A second informal workshop on ethnography with Elijah Anderson, Mabel Berezin, Renée Fox, Demi Kurz, Robin Leidner,

and Victoria Smith inspired me to spend as much time as I do discussing qualitative methods and their problems.

The aid of colleagues elsewhere was invaluable. Joel Frader has
been generous with his time over the years. His knowledge of both
pediatrics and bioethics saved me countless embarrassing mistakes. Robert Arnold saved me from a too-simplistic reading of physician autonomy. Steve Hilgartner and Mark Jacobs provided a
careful reading of the text at a critical point. Barry Schwartz provided helpful commentary to several chapters. An invitation from
Carol Heimer to speak at an American Sociological Association
meeting got me working on fieldnotes long filed away. A long and
critical but very helpful critique from an anonymous reviewer for
the University of Chicago Press was a spur to deal directly with
many of the issues that an earlier draft handled obliquely.

Fai Coffin, Carol Gardner, Penny Jeannechilde, Barbara Waxman,
and Valerie Root Wolpe helped with fieldnote transcriptions at early
stages of the project. Deborah Putnam Thomas, whose patience
and eyesight were strained through multiple revisions, made the
production of the text possible. Together, we worried about the de-
forestation necessary to bring this book to completion.

Finally, my wife, Marjorie, as always, read each word that I wrote
with care and insisted, as always, that garbled prose could never be
good sociology. More importantly, she used her clinical skills to
help me overcome my reluctance to deal with the interpersonal issues raised by genetic counseling. Her sense of humor and proportion sustained me through the writing and rewriting of this book.
My daughters, Emily and Abigail, were a constant reminder of my
own good fortune as I wrote about the painful experiences of other
parents not as blessed.

It goes without saying that the faults, mistakes, and problems that
remain are solely my responsibility.

INTRODUCTION

In the waning years of the 1970s, when I began this study of genetic counseling, I was unaware of the fact that this medical specialty existed and equally unaware of what workers in it did. Before entering the field, my first, untutored response was one of horror at the specter of the "brave new world" that an enterprise like genetic counseling promised. As a professional social scientist and as an ethnographer, I knew I had to neutralize the melodramatic quality of that first response in order to be an unbiased observer. My job, as I saw it, was to view genetic counseling as consisting of ordinary, recurrent transactions between a set of servers and a set of people who sought their service—a typical professional-client dyad.

This was very difficult to do. Somehow, I was overwhelmed by the enormity of the kinds of decisions that parents had to make. I was overwhelmed as well by the neonatal intensive care unit. I had trouble coming face to face with the various forms that genetic defects take; observing physical exams was always a personal trial. In addition, I was troubled by a sense of the incommensurable. What I observed, what I recorded was so prosaic; yet the implications of advances in genetic science, which promise to revolutionize medical practice, are anything but ordinary.

I never fully resolved that sense of distance between what I saw and what it all might mean. The text concentrates on what I saw. I followed a program that I devised from the work of Everett

C. Hughes for understanding genetic counselors, a program that concentrated on workplace routines, everyday understandings, and normal operating procedures. With Hughes as my guide, I sought a strategy for doing the fieldwork that would allow me to use the local knowledge that I gathered more generally. The strategy I adopted can be expressed as four commandments.

The First Commandment: Immerse yourself in the workgroup's everyday life—its repetitive, predictable troubles, its manner of coping with them, its sense of mastery, its experiences of defeat, its shared language for understanding its mission.

The Second Commandment: Study the workgroup's most naturally recursive activities, especially its routines, emergencies, and mistakes; describe what workers do and say to whom, under what conditions, in these three situations.

The Third Commandment: Dramaturgically describe behaviors as solutions to universally recurrent problems of the human condition—the riddles and persistent paradoxes that inhere in a collective life.

The Fourth Commandment: Always follow this interpretive injunction when assessing self-interested claims: Humble the proud, and elevate the humble.

It is this last injunction that makes genetic counselors a particularly instructive group for the student of professionals. They are a proud group—medical professionals—who in some sense have already been humbled. They refer to themselves as a mop-up service in their moments of exasperation; they feel overloaded by dirty work created by their colleagues' awkwardness; they are unable to preserve their own workday agendas and professional autonomy, for they have no "real," "genuine" treatment emergencies, no life-and-death decisions to make. They are called upon frequently, however, to consult at the bedside with colleagues who do have such emergencies, and the counselors find it gratifying both to be needed and to help.

The genetic counselors I studied were all physicians, but this is now rarely the case. One might even argue that the proud task of genetic counseling has been humbled, as it is now routinely carried out by workers of lesser prestige in the hospital hierarchy than physicians. But whether they graduate from medical school or come to the field by some alternative pathway, genetic counselors define themselves as professionals, define their core task as risk-assessment, and adopt generally, as a matter of professional ideology, a nondirective stance.

As professionals, genetic counselors are a sociological paradox: they are professionals whose knowledge base is as complex and abstract as any imaginable, yet they have virtually no power or autonomy. The genetic counselor's work is in the wings but not far from the footlights of hospital action (Goffman 1967). They are information specialists, neutral staters of odds, problem experts, decision facilitators rather than decision makers. They perform socially enabling work for clients who are either other medical professionals or lay persons. To follow the Hughesian program was socially enabling for me; it focused my attention on what genetic counselors did, for whom, in what circumstances.

This in turn raised different questions about the professional-client dyad. These questions are old-fashioned in two senses. First, they clearly describe a time past when the doctor-patient relationship was more primal in the hospital, when the professional server-client-user relationship was not of the interest it is now to so many third parties, and when the applications of genetics to clinical medicine were less complex. Second, these questions have in them faint echoes of classical sociological theory. For example, there are questions that have their roots in the writings of German sociologist Max Weber: Are the genetic counselors perfect, value-neutral experts who have embraced science as a vocation? Is this a part of a dreaded but promised "iron cage"? Is this what the disenchantment of the world looks like? Are genetic counselors "specialists without spirit, sensualists without heart" (Weber 1958, 182)? There are questions that have their roots in the French sociologist Émile Durkheim: Is genetic counseling the kind of ceremony that one would expect in a society where the cult of the individual prevailed and the collective conscience was diffuse, attenuated, and abstract? Are genetic counseling specifically and medical care more generally examples of the bureaucratization, routinization, and secularization of experience in modern society, indices of the withering of the sacral and the mysterious? There are questions that have their roots in Simmel: Is genetic counseling the form that help and care take in a society dominated by a spirit of calculation? Is genetic counseling for clients a manifestation of one of the forms that the blasé attitude takes in modern urban life?

These questions should all be understood as background concerns against which I carried out my empirical inquiry. They should also signal the kind of work this is: an empirically informed, theoretical speculation about the nature of professional service that is routinely dispensed in the pediatric hospital. Genetic counselors are used in this discussion as figures of social speech in two ways common to ethnographic writing: synecdoche and metaphor. Synecdoche, because a part, the transactions of a small, nonrepresentative group (genetic counselors) is used to represent a more complex, variegated whole: the medical profession. Metaphor, because the types of encounters they have with their clients and patients will be seen as exemplars of and for professional service in the modern state.

However, the use of a Hughesian framework to understand the work of genetic counselors defeats the downtrodden. It also presents a stylistic problem in ethnographic draftsmanship. How does one humble the proud when the proud think of themselves as a medical mop-up service? At the same time, taking the modest claims of genetic counselors at face value and letting the data speak for itself has problems all its own, for it misses much of what is disturbing about routine genetic services. Describing a knife-edge, present ethnography runs the risk of slicing off the past and future.

With routine genetic services, it is important to remember the past. Terrible things have been done in the past under the rubric of routine genetic policy. But this is a different time, a different place. The fact that Tay-Sachs screening is generally the model for successful voluntary community screening (Kaback 1977) shows how much this is so. However, neither the "Progressive Era's" genetic practice with regard to the congenitally feeble-minded (Gould 1981; Haller 1963; Reilly 1987), nor the racial and genetic assumptions behind the Tuskegee Syphilis Study (Jones 1981), nor those behind the interment of Japanese Americans in special centers (Drinnon 1986) reassure us about the strength of the barrier American jurisprudence creates to abuses based on so-called genetic thinking.

Further, to look at genetic counseling from its most concentrated technical base, the pediatric hospital, reduces the complexity of the fundamental social problems with which genetic counselors deal to a medical frame. But it is important to see in the organization of care new solutions to recurrent problems embedded more broadly in collective life. Communities, either at a state or local level, have had to deal with severely damaged neonates or with the question of whose genes are allowed to mix with whose. At a communal level, there was a time when not providing treatment for a deformed Jewish male until after the *bris* (ritual circumcision) was an outlawed, if furtively followed, medical practice. At a state level, antimiscegenation laws were enacted to protect gene pools, much as segregation kept the water clean in public ones. Genetic screening of newborns for rare metabolic diseases, voluntary carrier testing for sickle-cell anemia, Tay-Sachs disease, and thalassemia, "Baby Doe" regulations—these are all abstracted, post-modernist algorithms for older more primitive formulas.

These newer algorithms are represented here as a set of shop-floor actions, in order to provide dynamic explanations of how life-and-death judgments become banal routines in medical and professional work. But a humdrum banality was not what I originally imagined myself describing. Dramatic advances in fetal and neonatal diagnosis and treatment define medical frontiers, and it is to such frontiers, from the neonatal intensive care unit to fetal surgery, that the sociological ethnographer is often drawn. It was where I wanted to be. Unfortunately, it was not where the genetic counselors were. When such dramatic medical action unfolded, the genetic counselors were involved as extras. If they had any role to play at all in such situations, members of the counseling team were there to mop up after the medical crisis.

As an ethnographer seeking medical action, I was Ishmael on the wrong boat. In what follows, I hope to convey a sense of the terrible ordinariness of genetic counseling as an everyday activity. Yet despite my awareness of the dreary work routines associated with the practices of genetic counselors, I never fully worked through a fundamental and futile opposition to the very idea of genetic treatment. I cannot explain this. It is in an irrational sentiment that, try as

I might, I cannot silence. I do not know why, but this moral qualm feels like a failing to be an impartial, objective sociological observer.

In the final analysis, long after the immediacy of being in the field has faded, I remain disturbed by the fact that the everyday practice of genetics was so unobjectionable in the early 1980s and that it remains largely unobjectionable today. As Troy Duster argues, the scientific practice of genetics by physicians in the community in its most benign form keeps open a *Backdoor to Eugenics* (Duster 1990). Recent developments only pry the back door open wider. The normative question—How can this be done?—continues to trouble me even though the empirical one—How is it done?—is no longer much of a mystery or source of deep concern.

The fact that this back door is ajar worries me, as does the hubris of the enterprise. The mapping of the human genome, the prenatal screening of fetuses for genetic fitness, the therapeutic manipulation of our genetic make-up—all of these are audacious exercises, even if they are also part of a Kuhnian normal science. I cannot tell which is the greater hubris, that we try to do all these things, that we do them with so few second thoughts, or that we do them despite the magnitude of second thoughts.

I was narrowly educated within a classical canon. Hubris is a foreshadowing of tragedy. In American society such anxieties about the limits of activism and meliorative intervention are all too difficult to express and easy to discount. Once we can do something, it is generally too late to ask if we want to, or where we wish to stop. As an ethnographer stuck in a banal present, I found it difficult to fashion out of the flow of everyday activity, out of everyday discourse about probabilities, out of the ongoing interactional routines of genetic counselors, the deep cultural questions raised by the growing ascendance of "genetic reasoning" in American culture. In the field, I would have no trouble heeding the injunction, "Let sleeping dogs lie." But at a remove, as an ethnographer at a desk, the injunction loses its force. I have trouble precisely locating the larger cultural questions in the ongoing work of genetic counselors and those who consult them, and I have to ask, Why?

Watching the counselors work, it is hard to make any connection at all between past abuses of genetics and the practice of the genetic counselors I observed. Counselors are so called to signal the patient voluntarism at the heart of the contemporary practice of genetics as opposed to prior state-mandated eugenic efforts, to mark the difference between abuse and proper scientific practice of genetics (Reed 1974; Ludmerer 1972).

Genetic counseling as a service is generally a matter of transferring information to individuals who request it, and then leaving those individuals alone to make the tragic choices based on that information. This concern for individual privacy is an important part of the work ideology of genetic counselors. Patient autonomy is the bedrock of virtually all authoritative statements about the professional practice of genetics (Fraser 1974, Rosenstock, Childs, and Simopoulous 1975). So it is not surprising to discover that as genetic counselors do their work, they adopt a nondirective stance. Moreover, this is not even much of a discovery, since this is what, when first surveyed, genetic counselors say they do (Sorenson and Cuthbert 1979). In all of medical practice, it is hard to imagine a more prosaic activity performed with better intention than genetic counseling. Nonetheless, it is necessary to examine how this neutrality works rather than to simply accept the workers' statements that they practice it.

It is much easier to describe the practice of genetic counselors than to identify what is troubling in this, all the more so since exquisite, almost miraculous, and certainly breathtaking technical competence is a central feature of clinical genetic services. Of course, this breathtaking technical competence itself is based on a number of rather routine tasks: the penetration of a woman's abdomen with a needle for amniocentesis, the cutting and pasting of a photograph of a cell into a karyotype (a picture of a chromosome taken through a microscope). But nonetheless, however ordinary the process by which it is done, there was something miraculous about photographing genes in the early 1980s. Since this research was done, the number of mundanely accomplished miracles of modern science has only grown. Yet there is something disturbing about the way genetics is applied, something resonant with much of what is so wrong with medical practice as a human service more generally. Troubling yet paradoxical, for the problem seems to be one of goals realized: the physician could not be a better technical expert, the patient could not be granted any greater autonomy. There is so much effort, so much expense, so much time, and so much trouble, yet there is little gain and so much perduring existential pain.

All ethnography becomes social history. As time passes, a description of the way things are quickly becomes an account of the way things were. This fieldwork was done ten years ago. Much has changed in applied human genetics as I brooded about how to describe it. New technologies have made for increasingly refined diagnoses of *in utero* defects. Fewer physicians have pursued careers as genetic counselors. The task has been largely taken over by genetic associates. This fission in the medical division of labor is part of a general trend to shift mundane tasks to less specialized and less expensive workers. Prenatal testing, then a relatively rare and specialized service, has become a much more routine part of obstetric care. Genetic counseling is often bundled into obstetric practice in the form of standard and well-documented risk disclosures.

These changes in the structural arrangements of genetic counseling notwithstanding, the process of counseling appears static. Being able to identify this or that defect on the short arm of chromosome 4, which was previously not discoverable, may mean a great deal to a couple faced with having a child with this now-preventable defect. Whether a genetic associate or a physician discloses this news to them may have some bearing. But the way the information is transferred, how decision-making responsibility is allocated, and what issues are considered as part of the calculus for exercising responsibility—all of these appear unchanged. As medical professionals, genetic counselors take other people's emergencies and fashion out of them their own work routines, which is what Hughes long ago claimed professionals did.

The ethnographic description is meant to work at multiple levels. On the one hand, I am describing a specific moment in the development of a medical area of specialization—the moment just before and immediately following the United States Public Health Services' declaration "that mid-trimester amniocentesis is an accurate and highly safe procedure that does not add significant risk to the pregnancy" (Love, Alexander, Bryla, and Seigel 1978). On the other hand, I describe some recurrent problems that health professionals face when they attempt to apply their expertise to help patients: uncertainty, impotence, and the limits of rational mastery —issues that are at the core of medical sociology. Over and over again, I will invoke that marvelous phrase of Everett C. Hughes, "the rough edge of professional practice." Ultimately, that edge is the space where the patient's unique tragedy meets with the professional's everyday routines.[1] However, I will have little to say about the patient's side of this rough edge, although I will comment in chapter 7 on my retreat from patients and their problems. Instead, I shall concentrate on the worker's side of the edge to show how repetitive work routines dull it.

The empirical descriptions, then, are a mixture of the past and present, of the ephemeral and the unchanging in dispensing professional service: an ethnography and a commentary on ethnography. The first and last chapters deal with the problematics of the fieldwork. In the others, I describe the work of genetic counseling as a bundle of workplace demands from colleagues and clients. I try to bring to life a set of "good people engaged in dirty work." I am amblyopic—I would not mention this were it not such a good metaphor for the text, and were not the debate over the source of this defect (my mother's or my father's side of the family) such a good example of what happens in so many families with more serious defects to account for. One eye is pressed on matters close at hand; the other is focused on the distance. One eye observes; the other observes the observing.

This text begins with a discussion of problems I faced as an ethnographer invited into a setting to provide help. When I begin to provide an extensive discussion of their work activity in chapter 2, I will provide a detailed description of the cast of characters who

1. There is a problem in labeling those who see a counselor as *patients*. Most of these people are not ill. In designating them as patients, I am following the workplace practices of my subjects. This, of course, has problems of its own: namely, it reifies the view of reproduction as a medical problem that is inherent in genetic counseling.

make up the counseling team. I need here to supply enough background for readers to understand something about the setting into which chapter 1 plunges them.

Nightingale Children's Center is a 312-bed, level-3 pediatric facility. It provided state-of-the-art care and training in both general pediatrics and all of the pediatric subspecialties. Its level-3 designation indicated that as a regional center, the most complex pediatric problems elsewhere would be transferred to its wards. Nightingale's fame as a clinical center was matched by its reputation as a scientific research center. In addition, Nightingale Children's Center was a focus of local pride and philanthropy—a proud symbol of what the urban community in which it was nestled was willing to do for its children in need.

Nightingale Children's Center has been described elsewhere in better detail than I can provide. The omission of proper crediting by a footnote here is intentional; it is to preserve anonymity. This bare mention is a compromise in the conflict between the norms of scholarship and those of fieldwork.

Among the divisions of Nightingale Children's Center was the clinical genetics center. Attached to this unit were physicians who did the work of genetic counseling as well as the personnel of a cytogenetics laboratory which analyzed the results of amniocenteses and carried out basic research.

The genetic counselors at Nightingale were all physicians; this makes them somewhat different from genetic counselors who are not, but are the products of relatively recently created programs in genetic counseling. Counseling itself is provided in a clinic that is utilized on different times and days for different specialties. As a result, treatment rooms are devoid of any decoration; the waiting area has no amenities such as reading materials. The impersonality of the setting is in sharp contrast to the personal type of service that is supposed to be provided, which is conveyed by the label *counseling*.

Were this an account which had as its objective the most representative portrait of genetic counseling possible, any case study would be utterly inadequate. However, the goal of this account is somewhat different. While I seek to provide an account of the work of genetic counselors—a description of the services they provide both to patients and physician colleagues—I seek as well to look at the management of clinical authority in a pediatric hospital and to use the counselors as my entrée. For this task, the counselors are an ideal choice. They do not exercise clinical authority. Nonetheless, they possess an advantage all their own, for when a contest over autonomy is staged, extras are called in early. As part of the counseling crew, I got to watch, but from a distance.

At another level, this is a book about the delivery of professional services. One admittedly atypical group of doctors is pressed into service in a case study of how the responsibilities and obligations of medical professionals are defined in the modern hospital. Nonetheless, some of the phenomena I describe (the worker's ability to take momentous events and render them routine and prosaic, the reduction of complex moral issues to technical questions, and the manipulation of patient autonomy by physicians as a sword to compel some decisions and as a shield to avoid responsibility for others) are useful starting points for a thick description of what genetic counseling is—a thick description of a slim encounter with yet another helping professional.

While I certainly realize how genetic counselors differ from all other medical and health professionals, I want to highlight the problematics at the core of applying service rationales at all. In particular, I want to concentrate on those areas where our ability to explain, to diagnose, and to describe outruns our ability to help. So there is a double focus in speaking about genetic counselors. I am speaking about genetic counseling as a service and genetic counseling as an activity of professionals. Always the conduct described is meant to stand as an instance of action performed under an obligation of professional service. The descriptions themselves are mindful of how manipulable a claim of service is. The portrait of a working group starts with the most mundane, taken-for-granted activities. We begin with clinical routines and move on to hospital emergencies; then we end with more problematic exercises of authority.

There has been a recurrent tension in producing this ethnography. This tension is an interpretive one: when to focus on the concrete interaction and when to look beyond it for broader cultural significance. I want to describe both the Blakean heaven in a single grain of sand and to use these particles to contribute to the ongoing discourse about the workplace, about service, and about communication with professional information specialists.

In so doing, I have in mind two distinct audiences. The first is fellow sociologists and ethnographers. For them, this is meant as a discussion of the hospital as a professional shop, a meditation on some of the difficulties in doing ethnographic work, and an analysis of some of the mistakes I made doing this research. The second audience comprises those involved with medical humanities, bioethics, or applied medical ethics. For them, I hope the text is data, discussion material for these new medical professionals involved in resolving the complex questions that surround care in the modern hospital.

Trying to please two audiences is never easy. The philosophizing on ethnography may appear defensive to those outside sociology, untroubled by the debates inside the field about how this activity is best done. The discussion of ethical matters may appear overly moralizing to sociologists trained, as I was, to look at social life as it is, not as we might wish it to be. I studied a marginal professional group with a methodology only marginally acceptable in my discipline, however much it is appreciated outside sociology. The ethnography, like the organized practice of genetics, organizes marginality.

One further comment on moralizing is necessary before wading into the text. Although not realized in the present, there is the potential of tragic scenarios, of a genetic dystopia, as we follow our inclination to tinker with ourselves. These, however, are products of theoretical speculation, not empirical investigation, and they are the source of much commentary elsewhere (Suzuki and Knudtson 1990). There are also recurrent, personal tragedies at the everyday level. For while genetic counseling does not remedy many problems, it does, through therapeutic abortions, save some individuals from the burdens and pains of raising offspring with devastating and overwhelming problems. When I began this project, I saw decisions following positive amniocentesis as simple matters—as admitting only one right choice—for any rational decision maker armed with a utilitarian calculator. Now I no longer do so, although I long for the moral certainty I once had. What I have tried to do in this volume is capture the context that makes, as Hippocrates once noticed, "decision difficult." That decisions are difficult should come as no surprise. How to allocate miserable choices is always a problem in group life. What I did not realize was how hard it would be to imagine one part of "birthwork" as separate from all the rest; how difficult it would be to see genetic counseling as an individual piece of a system of medical care.

1

INVITATION
TO ETHNOGRAPHY

What should couples with Huntington's chorea do about childbearing? What do genetic counselors advise them to do? Are there genetic grounds for compelling a couple to have a so-called therapeutic abortion? How are birth defects explained to parents who bear children with these defects? In this volume, I shall report on how these problems were managed in one workgroup: a genetic counseling team in an elite urban medical center. These observations are the empirical basis for a sociological discussion of problems in applying new technologies of prenatal monitoring and diagnosis. They serve as well as a springboard for considering the rights and responsibilities, duties and obligations embedded in role relationships.

I collected the primary data during two intensive periods of participant observation among a team of genetic counselors who invited me to join them because they were aware that the services they offered patients were bound to involve questions of a social sort.[1] These services included counseling couples who either al-

1. The invitation to observe came in the spring of 1976. Preliminary observation lead to a proposal which was subsequently funded by the National Institute of Child Health and Development. The first period of intense observation began in the fall of 1976 and ended in the winter of 1978. In the winter of 1980, I reentered the field, only to leave again in mid-autumn of that year. My comings and goings were not random or unmotivated, but were rationalized theoretically at the same time that they were personally necessary. For now, that is all that needs to be said about the matter. The confessional of the fieldworker (Van Maanen 1988) is more appropriately an appendix to a text than a sentence in a footnote.

ready had, or were believed to be at risk for having, a genetically defective offspring, as well as diagnostic testing. At the time of observation, no treatments for defects discovered *in utero* were available. The fact that this has changed and that for some rare deformities fetal surgery is possible only intensifies those questions of "a social sort."

As a result of the counselors' invitation, I joined their workgroup. I attended preclinic conferences at which management of upcoming cases was discussed, observed the counseling sessions themselves, and listened to the counselors evaluate their work in a postclinic conference. In addition, I interviewed a sample of parents whose counseling sessions I had attended in order to gather their understanding of the process. Finally, I was on call for those emergency situations in which physicians in the newborn nursery or the neonatal intensive care unit needed to consult with the physicians specializing in clinical genetics.

The interactional data from my first-hand observations is the starting point for each discussion of shopfloor work. But to write of genetic counselors ethnographically is not to write of some tribe isolated in the bush, impervious to the wider world around them. Both genetic counselors and sociological observers who trail behind them need to take that wider world into account. Ethnographic descriptions of the applications of clinical genetics in the modern American hospital need to be mindful of the legacy of earlier attempts at eugenics, as well as the legal, political, and cultural questions that current practices raise.[2]

Starting with interactional data, the lived experience of patients and their doctors, I will move beyond thick description (Geertz 1976) to an analysis of what these patterns of interaction say about role systems, their domains, and their boundaries; about areas of

2. The introduction briefly considered historical antecedents of current attempts at applying genetic knowledge. In assessing current attempts at applied eugenics, we need to consider as well contemporary attitudes about risk, technology, the nature of birth, and therapeutic abortion. In trying to parse the current meaning of clinical genetics, the behavioral events observed have little meaning outside their arenas of production and interpretation. Some areas of genetics have become social problems, while others are relatively unproblematic. Understanding why this is so is a major task of the sociology of social problems (Hilgartner and Bosk 1988; Schneider 1985).

collective consensus, uncertainty, or confusion; and about the policy alternatives we face as a collectivity.

An Invitation to Fieldwork

I was invited into this setting as a guest of the genetic counseling team because of their sense that as a sociologist trained to observe behavior as it naturally occurs, I would have something useful to add about how best to manage the myriad of social problems that trailed in the wake of new clinical developments. Since professional groups so rarely invite study by outsiders, it is first necessary to comment, albeit briefly, on this invitation and its implications for the ethnography before moving on to the substance of the text.

I received this invitation because I am a medical sociologist, an ethnographer of medical action. Here it is worth mentioning that today I would be unlikely to receive such an open-ended invitation. Since this fieldwork was done, formal institutions (ethics committees) and workers (bioethicists) have emerged for managing precisely the types of issues that the genetic counselors wanted help with. Back then, it was not so, and the help of any ethnographer was sought. By any technical, formal, scientific criterion, my data-gathering techniques are primitive, crude, and inevitably interlaced with my own subjectivity. I observe patients, physicians, and nurses as they go about the business of being ill, curing, and caring. My data comprises the behaviors I observe, the conversations I overhear, and the responses to questions I am not too timid to ask. At a phenomenological level alone, being a medical ethnographer is a peculiar occupation. For example, fieldwork on a genetic counseling service involves repeated voluntary participation in and observation of many of life's most awful moments, watching others cope with what the genetic counselors, ruefully echoing those who seek their services, refer to as "all God's mistakes."

However odd the work, anthropologists in the bush and sociologists on urban streetcorners have made ethnography a familiar mode of academic discourse. For the ethnographer in a medical setting, health-care workers are an exotic tribe; the bounded whole of the modern hospital is the bush. Our task is to report on the goings-on in this faraway province. At worst, we are voyeurs whose

reports are a source of academic cheap thrills; at best, we are witnesses reporting on the most profound dilemmas of the human
condition.

Not surprisingly, I prefer the latter self-description. As witnesses,
we have two objectives. The first is to provide an empirically thick
description of what happened: who did what, to whom, in what circumstances, with what responses from others, to what end, and
with what consequences. The second is to analyze this description
of the everyday, ordinary business of being a provider or consumer
of health services. We inspect the record, as it were, for the evidence it contains about what it means to be a person, a family member, a citizen in modern American society.

As a witness in the arena of everyday medical life, as a sociologist,
my perspective is explicitly dramaturgical. I think of clinical action
in terms of situations—in particular those in which clinical action is
problematic. Procedurally, I examine these situations to uncover
what rhetoric, rationales, maxims, myths, data, and bottom lines
physicians arm themselves with when they recommend one course
rather than another to patients, when they explain unexpected, unwanted outcomes, and when they search for reasons to explain
pain and suffering.[3]

As a medical sociologist/ethnographer, I have spent time in a variety of settings. However the settings varied, the central feature of
my work as a sociological ethnographer remained the same. Data
were generated by my skill at manipulating my relationship with
my subjects. Invariably, and at one level, ethnographers treat their
subjects simply as means to the end of generating good data on how
some intractable problem of the human condition is managed
among a group of natives.

Ethnographers—to the degree that they think about this practice
at all—justify it by sleight-of-hand. It is not particular people that we
are interested in, but general types, diffuse social and institutional
processes, or native understandings. If people are treated as a
means to an end, it is not *qua* people, but as mere representations

3. This paragraph is an echo of Garfinkel's (1967) charge for the study of social life
in "What Is Ethnomethodology?" The echo is meant as a gesture of respect and a
literal description of how I try to frame situations that are meaningful to me as a
medical sociologist who works methodically as an observer.

of categorical schema. In presenting data, we do not betray individual trusts and confidences; instead we generalize them.

Most fieldworkers are not invited into medical settings; they are more commonly self-invited guests, who find themselves backstage in medical arenas after complex negotiations to win institutional sanction. Most contemporary accounts of doctor-watching offered by sociologists stress the difficulties in gaining access to the private arenas in which medical activity takes place and in gaining the trust of physicians and other medical personnel. Fieldworkers invest the medical profession with many of the features that the nineteenth-century German sociologist Georg Simmel attributed to secret societies; then they describe themselves as minor Promethean figures eager to snatch secrets and place them in the public domain. In the most vulgar of fieldwork imagery, the medical profession is a living, breathing exemplar of G. B. Shaw's famous "conspiracy against the laity." The sociologist's task is to expose this conspiracy for what it is—the exploitation of pain and vulnerability for profit.

In characterizing the relations of doctors and patients, conflict is the social process and hostility is the emotional tone that are most frequently highlighted. Most medical ethnographer's heed Hughes' (1971) injunction to study the "rough edges" of medical practice, those areas where lay and professional expectations about what action is necessary are least likely to converge. It is tempting to interpret this focus as the result of the difficulties experienced in gaining access to the fieldwork setting.

But what happens when such resistance is absent? What happens when the fieldworker does not worm his or her way into a site to pursue a personal agenda, but is invited in by physicians who have their own version of what the ethnographer's task is and what it ought to be?

Most practically, I experienced none of the difficulties associated with gaining entrance to the field setting. There were no negotiations with hospital administrators, no multiple clearances from multiple clinicians, and no endless rounds of meetings to explain who I was and what I was about. I was never asked to make elaborate promises to safeguard the confidentiality and anonymity of the institution or its physicians. Never was there any suggestion that my work be subject to any sort of prepublication preview. I had to obtain the official approval of an institutional review board, but that had more to do with government policy toward research subjects than with physicians' distrust of fieldworker sociologists. Moreover, as we shall see, I was asked by counselors on numerous occasions not to gather a consent but, nonetheless, to be in attendance.

Pilot observations began before the institutional approval was granted. Beyond that, the genetic counselors had been observed regularly by social scientists long before I got there. In the previous year, four graduate students had done fieldwork projects; one faculty member in the Law School came to clinic and conferences quite regularly; and finally, a fifth graduate student was making observations preliminary to a dissertation proposal. At the same meeting at which the group asked me to join them, they worried out loud about "chronic crowding and being overstudied."

Of course, the absence of obstacles, as well as the plethora of observers, spoke of the desire of genetic counselors to receive sociological help. Their invitation to me was yet another artifact of their desire to provide their services as sensibly as possible. When they approached me, genetic counselors were aware that they were providing a new clinical service that intersected with some highly charged areas of social life, including the nature of parenthood and family bonds, and the permissibility of, and limits to, an actively preventive eugenics. In addition, the genetic counselors stated that there "were bound to be other difficulties that they could not foresee."

They asked for my help, which they envisioned as taking two forms. First, I could perform a hard-headed, objective, assessment of how they were managing problems. In addition, I could provide a catalogue of the typical problems that they face but lack adequate resources to resolve. In accomplishing the first task, I would serve as an efficiency expert for the genetic counselors, providing data which allowed them to improve the quality of their services. In accomplishing the second, I would be a "committed moral entrepreneur," providing the society at large with data that would confirm the need to commit an even greater supply of resources to genetic counseling.

The genetic counselors believed that such a commitment was necessary and that, if I came to know their world as they did, I too would find such a need inescapable. This expectation—that our sentiments and analyses of societal interest would prove to be congruent—was, of course, unstated at the outset. It came with the invitation, but I did not realize it at the time.

At those early meetings, I was most struck by the counselor's recognition that the application of genetic knowledge in clinical situations created problems and that an interdisciplinary effort was called for to resolve them. I eagerly accepted the counselors' invitation, unaware of the implications of being invited to join the team—unaware of the difference between being an invited guest and being, as is more typically the case for a medical sociologist, an uninvited, albeit tolerated intruder. Flattered by the idea that I might be useful, that I might have something to offer, I was seduced by the idea of pseudo-colleagueship. Not aware of the way this invitation, which amounted, after all, to nothing more than an opportunity to be an unpaid consultant, was a subtle devaluing of social science expertise, I joined the group. I joined unmindful of the consequences that belonging might have, first for observation, and later for reporting.

Invited Guests and Uninvited Intruders

If invited guest/uninvited intruder was a status distinction of which I was initially unaware, I quickly learned many of its nuances. In previous work, I had been an uninvited intruder (Bosk 1979). As such, I felt no special loyalties to the groups that I studied. I felt all the ordinary social constraints to treat them and their world with decency and respect, but I also recognized that in the course of things, I would bruise their cherished notions of their own goodness. But that was all part of making the latent manifest, of looking at social life unsentimentally, of revealing what goes on backstage. It was a part of all the formulas that sociologists have constructed to describe the unique perspective on the human condition that ethnography provides.

As an uninvited intruder, my relationships with my subjects were complex. On the one hand, in my day-to-day interactions, my subjects had no expectations of me. I was ornamental, decorative, extraneous, and dispensable. If I kept out of the way, if I was marginally helpful, if I filled rare down-time with interesting talk, whatever I wrote later was my own business. On the other hand, I was constantly tested, made the butt of group jokes, and accepted very slowly in the setting. What is critical is that whether I was an object of disinterest or suspicion for my subjects, I was expected to contribute nothing fundamental to the ongoing life of the group. When I did help, when I opened packages, passed supplies, or was simply an extra pair of hands, it was a welcome surprise to the surgeons. Expectations were low, and satisfying them was easy.

This was not the case when I was an invited guest. The genetic counselors had invited me to observe because they thought that I might help them. This expectation to be useful was unfamiliar to me. At case conferences, I was asked to provide concrete data about such things as how class differences or family structure affect patient understanding. I was asked to speculate about the handling of cases—to participate in the making of policy. How should couples who come in for sex selection be treated? What should the center's position on counseling for exposure to Agent Orange be?

Most frequently, the counselors asked for help on a range of clinical management issues: what social information to collect routinely for genetic registries, how best to give incoming patients reasonable expectations about their upcoming visit to the genetic counselor, how to avoid no-shows on clinic day, how to decide which patients needed which level of follow-up care, and so on.

It is Friday afternoon, late in the fall. I am sitting, as I do every Friday afternoon, in a conference room for the postclinic wrap-up session that members of the genetic counseling team hold to report on their counseling sessions. Al Samuels (all names have been changed) is reporting on a case. Samuels characterized the session as "strange." He could not get a "fix" on whether or not the couple understood what he told them.

He emphasized that they appeared to take everything, yet as the information got worse and worse, their affect did not change. Samuels giggled nervously as he concluded.

Berger, chief of the Service, asked Samuels if he knew

the parents' jobs. Samuels did not. Berger was displeased. He told the group that this was "standard medical information which should be on record." He added a sentence or two about the importance of this kind of data, and the group moved on to discuss other cases.

When the meeting broke up, I found myself going through the doorway with Berger. He led me a few paces away from the rest of the group and said, "I wish you'd push a little for medical records to include more social information. When I do, I sound just like a mother hen. But you, because you're a social scientist, perhaps you could get the others to see how important it is."

It was, of course, Berger who had initially invited me to join the workgroup. Here was a direct example of him telling me how he expected me to be useful, what he wanted me to do: Be a missionary for social science data on medical records. Other members of the team also felt entitled to make special requests of my services as an observer.

The Mulroneys are coming to clinic for counseling.[4] They have a child with tuberous sclerosis. Mrs. Mulroney is pregnant. All the members of the counseling team save Berger are convinced that Mr. Mulroney has an extraordinarily mild expression of tuberous sclerosis. Berger is convinced that Mr. Mulroney is normal, and to the horror of the group, he intends to counsel the couple that they are not at any increased risk for having an affected child.

Bill Smith calls me at my office. "Bosk, you comin' to clinic?" I tell him I am. "Good, we want you to sit in on the Mulroneys and tell us what Berger says. We all think he's close to a serious error. But he won't listen to anybody. We want to know what happens."

This request—to monitor a colleague—was the most frequent special request that the counselors made of me. I was used in this way quite often when there was disagreement at Wednesday's preclinic

4. For further discussion of the Mulroneys and their problems, see chapter 2.

conference about how to counsel the cases coming in that Friday. Not infrequently, I would be asked in postclinic conference if pre-clinic understandings were implemented, although never so nakedly as that. More often, it was just a vague invitation to talk: "Bosk, what did you think of the session?"

Conventionally, the sociological literature on fieldwork instructs us to turn such special requests and demands into occasions for educating our subjects about what fieldworkers do, or to volunteer just enough to get subjects to reveal their own feelings. The latter is a standard method for generating good field data.

With the genetic counseling team, neither approach was totally satisfactory. Didactic lectures *in situ* about the ethnographer's code of conduct and the importance of not interfering unduly with natu-rally occurring phenomena did not appear to be an adequate re-sponse to people who asked me to watch their work so that I could help. Moreover, even if I had wanted to help (and I am not certain that I did), more often than not I did not know how.

Called on often by the genetic counselors, I found that I had nothing particularly useful to say. Yet those invited to social occa-sions have obligations that those who merely intrude on them do not. As someone watching genetic counseling under the guise of having something instantly useful to offer, I often felt like a fraud when I let my hosts down by failing to meet their expectations.

I mention this because we shall see that my major criticism of the genetic counselors is their failure to be useful, to meet the patient on the patient's own ground, and to address the patient's most pressing concerns. The counselors, I will argue, at times use the goal of patient autonomy as a ground for patient abandonment. Sometimes, I wonder how much this insight grows out of my own sense of frustration at not being able to help the counselors more with applications of my specialist's knowledge in those very diffi-cult situations where my help was requested.

With this example, I wish to call attention to a similarity between the work of physicians and the medical sociologist who trails be-hind them. The work of both involves explaining imponderables, and the failure to do so occasionally feels like a failure to meet a moral obligation. This example is a miniparadigm of how I was taught to act as a fieldworker, to use my own responses in a situation as a guide to the responses of others.[5]

I have mentioned that I thought the genetic counselors used the ideal of patient autonomy as an excuse for patient abandonment.[6] This is a sharp criticism, and since sharp criticism is often socially unpleasant (the essence of sheer effrontery), such sharp criticisms present a special problem to those invited into fieldwork settings: how to voice them in a way that does not give offense.

To use a social analogy, I was often in the position of the guest invited for a dinner where the experience of the meal itself is the entertainment—a feast. For this guest, nothing has been spared. The host has set the table with the best cutlery and china, given great attention to the menu, used the finest ingredients in preparing the dishes, and, nonetheless, produced an indifferent meal.

The guest is acutely aware of the meal's shortcomings; the host, however, is proud of his or her best effort. The meal consumed, the host turns toward the guest and awaits some comment. The host may grow anxious and fish for a response. The guest needs to find a way to respond to the feast that balances gratitude with honesty. That was my problem.

As hosts, the genetic counselors were unfailingly gracious. They offered me access to situations so acutely private that I sought rationales to limit my access. Gracious as hosts, the counselors were also anxious. They were constantly soliciting my evaluation of the fare they had placed before me.

Situations in which I had nothing to add presented me with one type of problem. My silence on troubling questions for me marked my failure to meet the moral and social obligations of the occasion

5. As a miniparadigm, it is a good example because it is so extreme, because it makes so much of the fieldworker's subjectivity, and because, like fieldwork itself, it is nonfalsifiable.

6. While I speak in this volume about genetic counselors first and foremost, I do not feel that counselors alone are guilty of using autonomy as a warrant for abandonment. I am not singling out counselors as the solitary abandoners of patients amongst all the medical profession. Instead, I am using counselors to show how rather extensive patient abandonment can occur under the banner of more perfect patient autonomy. The very fact that counselors can abandon patients is noteworthy because it runs counter to so many elements of their occupational ideology.

to which my hosts had invited me. Situations where negative commentary was unavoidable presented another. What was the best response, if a commentary was requested, when I felt (as was most rarely the case) that the counselors had badgered their clients, or (as was all too often the case) when I felt that counselors had abandoned their patients by evading the real patient issues.

On the one hand, I did not want to insult my hosts' hospitality. On the other, I did not want to respond enthusiastically to dismal fare, only to see it served up proudly on all occasions. What did I owe the genetic counselors as a result of the unique field opportunity that they afforded me? At one level, I felt that I owed it to them to present my criticisms at a very high level of generality, so that it was not individual counselors that I was criticizing, but the structural arrangements of care and the organization of social roles. But this satisfies the social obligation at a great remove from the time when it was actually incurred. How in the everyday context did I mix candor and kindness to respond to the needs of the genetic counselors?

The Witness Role

If I could be neither a garrulous nor an enthusiastic guest, in the spirit of the genetic counselors' invitation to join their team, what role then did I come to play in my three years with the counselors? How did I balance the genetic counselors' expectation that I be useful with my own methodological determination to remain detached and objective?[7]

I defined my work in two ways. I watched doctors with a well-defined set of sociological purposes at hand. I watched them to learn about the doctor-patient relationship, the division of labor, and the management of risk in the academic medical setting. But I also witnessed for doctors, and this witnessing for doctors was a more complicated business than ordinary sociological watching.

7. Another old-fashioned aspect of this account was my determination to remain value-neutral. This is a role that both sociologists and anthropologists have long ago abandoned for a more forthright advocacy for the disadvantaged or paid consultancy for the privileged. Aware of the development of a more clinical sociology, I find it hard now to explain why I struck such a distant and remote definition of the task at hand.

During the time I observed them, the genetic counselors faced many of the dilemmas that have become so familiar in the bioethics literature. For example, on several occasions the genetic counseling service debated whether children with trisomy 21 should be allowed to die from repairable defects; decided how the marginally competent mentally retarded should be presented with their reproductive choices; discussed whether parents were under any obligation to abort defective fetuses; speculated upon whether surrogate motherhood was a permissible remedy for certain forms of infertility (this well in advance of media disclosure and judicial notice of the practice); and tried to formulate cases under which amniocentesis for sex selection was ever acceptable practice. And this is only a partial list.

On many occasions, I was present not by chance but because my presence was specifically requested. Like the witness to any ceremony, my attendance was supposed to act as some sort of guarantee that proprieties were observed, that patient rights were respected, and that all the acceptable alternatives for resolving a problem had been explored. At the same time, I was a witness to the pain and suffering of patients as well as to how seriously the counselors took that pain and how hard they worked to mitigate it.

What separates witnessing for doctors from merely watching them with some well-directed set of academic purposes at hand is this: Witnessing seems more directed to establishing or ratifying a moral community than mere watching. Over time, I came to realize that not only did I witness for a group of physicians, but that those physicians did precisely the same for their patients. They listened to their patients pains and problems, and the fact of the listening confirmed that the suffering was real and legitimate. Providing a place far from neighbors, friends, and family for couples to talk with specialists was all by itself something of a service.

Hearing a physician raise the option of artificial insemination by donor as a way to lower the risk of recessive disorder, or hearing a physician raise the possibility of institutionalizing a profoundly retarded child or discuss the possibility of abortion after a positive amniocentesis did not mean that the couple would necessarily rush to utilize these options. But it did mean that they had permission to think about them and that to do so was not necessarily immoral. If they did not do anything specific for a patient's pain, genetic counselors, at the least, gave a place to take that pain; gave them "frames" and supplied "options." Given the shame and guilt that often accompany the birth of a damaged child, this was no small thing. Counselors then witnessed the pain of patients, and I witnessed the pain of counselors as they came face to face with their limitations in palliating the pains of their patients.

In a curious way, I came to symbolize for the group the moral community outside the hospital—my presence in highly problematic situations became a sign of approbation from the larger community of whatever course of action was taken. At one level this exacerbated my difficulties in giving the group negative feedback, but it resolved them at another. In any situation, I could simultaneously provide criticism and provide myself distance from it.[8] I would routinely speak not as an observer, but for some identifiable segment of the community and raise my objections in a voice that did not seem to be my own. I would begin most negative commentary by saying, "If I were a . . .", thus separating myself from my spoken words.

When the fieldworker is invited to join a medical team, witnessing is part of the fieldworker role at three different levels. First, at the simplest level, the fieldworker provides counselors with a "reality check," a confirmation that things are or were as they seemed. As a mundane example, whenever the genetic counselors described to others cases that I had observed, they would pepper their accounts with asides to me such as "Isn't that right?" or "That's what happened, isn't it?" Just as often, this confirmation was of the "God, did you see that?" variety; I helped make the incredible credible.[9]

Second, and unbeknownst to me at the time, a fieldworker, especially one whose presence has been requested, provides his subjects with a sense of legal protection. Being used this way happened to me late in my fieldwork, long after I had built upon that initial but

8. For a full development of role distance and the repertoire of techniques that surgeons and teen-age girls on carousels use to achieve it, see Goffman's (1961c) seminal essay. Here I am simply describing one ethnographer's ploy for achieving the same end.

9. Interestingly enough, I was used by surgeons in the same way. Some aspects of witnessing are built into the fieldworker role, whether the fieldworker is an invited guest or an intruder.

shallow trust that the genetic counselors extended with their invitation to observe. Rather commonly, I found myself being asked to observe cases which were complex and contested morally, bureaucratically, and legally. I was on a number of occasions asked to observe as a "working" member of the team, to forego obtaining an informed consent from subjects, and to desist from public note-taking. While it would have been both ethically safe (and correct) to refuse such offers, the actual situations, along with their attendant negotiations, were more complex than that. Did a refusal mean that I was unwilling to act as a member of the team? Did the counselors have the right to seek my aid this way? Did I have a duty to refuse?

The compromise we arrived at was to have me introduced as a sociologist working with the team. I did not take notes at the time of observation, but wrote the cases up from memory. When a lawyer came to gather data for a wrongful life case, whenever a couple sought amniocentesis for sex selection, whenever parents sought to withdraw treatment from neonates, the group could press me into service as a team member. I slowly came to realize—slowly, perhaps, because I was gathering such good data—that the genetic counselors expected that should the need arise, I could serve as an expert witness capable of stating what had really happened. I do not know why the discovery of this latent dimension of my fieldworker role surprised and disturbed me, but it did, despite the large role that expert witnesses play in the civil procedures of the society.[10] Moreover, I shared with my genetic counselor subjects the feeling that being called into service as a witness in this way was annoying and burdensome.[11]

Witnesses play a religious role as well. Like the rabbi at a slaughterhouse, the priest at an execution, or the airline chaplain who

10. Fieldworkers have long worried about being co-opted by those that they study, and this worry is all the greater when we are studying up the social structure rather than down. Empathy with the wretched in society is rarely, if ever, considered a methodological problem. On the other hand, empathy with the powerful, with physicians, is seen as considerable cause for alarm. Here, though, I am fretting about more than where my loyalties lay. I am concerned about what my expertise is as well: what does it mean to represent oneself as "a skilled ethnographer"; what, save writing skillful ethnographies, can others expect me to do?

11. See Bill Smith's comments about being a witness in a wrongful life action (chapter 5).

consoles those awaiting passengers on a flight that has crashed, they purify and sanctify messy situations. In allowing me to view their uncertainties, anxieties, and doubts, the genetic counselors had allowed me to see their group function in an intensely religious and spiritual way. In hearing the genetic counselors discuss birth, life, and death, the boundary between them, and the permissible limits of human intervention, I was a witness to the group's "collective meditation on sacred things." For those social scientists who take their Durkheim seriously, such a meditation is the essence of religious experience. As such, it tells something of what these medical professionals hold sacred.

As I have stated, the genetic counselors were all too aware of the ways in which the organization of genetic counseling might disturb lay sensibilities. Having as their only treatment recommendation second-trimester abortion, and practicing in a society where the right to perform this procedure was a hotly contested political issue, they could scarcely avoid the ethical tensions created by their work.[12] When most aware of these tensions, the counselors often tried to draw me into their deliberations as a medical ethicist. I invariably demurred when called on to act in this way. I mention this now only because my silence on matters of medical ethics as they unfolded in clinical situations is in such sharp contrast to my volubility in the pages below, which are so far removed from the contexts in which words might have been helpful.

Soft Data, Hard Problems

I also mention my silence regarding medical ethics because if fieldworkers' canons of methodological purity commit them not to act as situations unfold, then it seems fair to ask just what do they contribute; why are they there, and are they necessary? Most sim-

12. The genetic counselors have much in common with the abortion counselors described so well by Joffe (1987). There is, however, this important difference: The abortion counselors were guided by rationales anchored in an applied social utilitarianism. The genetic counselors were also applied utilitarians, but they anchored their utilitarianism in genetic knowledge and paid virtually no attention to the social and economic contexts of pregnancy. For the genetic counselors, the only unwanted pregnancies were those planned pregnancies in which the fetus had an identifiable defect.

ply, fieldworkers watch, listen, and use their own feelings and responses as guides to their interpretation of what is going on. In essence, this kind of observation is not terribly different from what psychiatrists, psychologists, and social workers are instructed to do as therapists. As Geertz (1976, 26) points out, ethnographic knowledge shares much with clinical inference.

The uniqueness of the fieldworker role comes from how that observation is used. Therapists are urged to use their feelings, instincts, and observations as a guide in responding to clients. For the therapist, for almost all those that use the logic of clinical diagnosis, the witnessing of action is a prelude to activity. This is true for other routine witnesses in the society as well, such as beat policemen and judges, basketball referees and baseball umpires, disability review panels and insurance adjusters.

This is not so for the fieldworker, who absorbs but does not respond to the situation. The task of the fieldworker is to witness again and again, but not to use the data gathered this way in interaction. Rather, the fieldworker observes to write. Patients, doctors, and most every other native ever observed, write as well. But unlike fieldworkers, they had to act; the fieldworker has only to observe. This freedom from intervention and from ordinary interaction allows fieldworkers their special purchase on social life.

Gusfield (1981) speaks of this purchase as an Olympian one. The image better describes the aspirations than the accomplishments of fieldworkers: namely, to describe without sentimentality the way the world works. The ethnographer produces a social description, which is an imaginative construct. This description unpacks the interlinkages between everyday understandings, power, authority, and routine social action in revealing why things are as they are. In addition, as Gusfield shows so masterfully in his analysis of drinking and driving, such a description provides a glimpse at alternative constructions of the social world.[13] Once the world is imagined in this way, it can be imagined differently.

13. Gusfield's analysis begins by questioning our collective conventional wisdom; for example, the taken-for-granted assumption that reducing the number of individuals who drink and drive is a policy lever for improving highway safety. Why, Gusfield asks, does not the lever lie elsewhere? He then identifies a number of plausible alternatives to conventional wisdom: improved mass transportation, safer

But what do sociologists as fieldworkers uniquely contribute to public life by imagining the world differently? This question has no simple answer. But if we return to the case of genetic counselors, we can provide a rough outline of the major dimensions of any adequate response to the question.

First, fieldwork alone places us in primary contact with social life as it is lived. The pains, the pressures, the perils, and the pleasures of the genetic counselor's work as well as the sorrow, shame, and existential guilt of parents are apprehended as they unfold in context, or are later commented on in soliloquies.[14] Fieldwork allows us to describe a set of fundamental life experiences as they occur— it provides us with words to inscribe the arc of human experience. In a field like genetic counseling, where the underlying technology threatens to revolutionize medical practice, it allows us to see the embedded tensions that lie beneath the surface of a rapidly advancing and dazzling medical technology: What is help? How is it provided in this society at this time? Fieldwork supplies precisely what other research methods drop out—the experiencing individual as a member of a community and the set of shared meanings that sustains that individual's action in an uncertain world. Fieldwork allows us to describe social life as we live it.

But that is not all fieldwork provides. It provides us with an opportunity not just to describe the lives we lead, but to analyze them. When it is performed with skill, it allows us to examine the shadow that falls between the image and the reality.[15] In the case of genetic counselors, this has meant matching counselors' statements about intent and purpose with daily encounters. For example, as we shall see in the next chapter, the counselors think of themselves as a sup-

highway design, more crash-worthy automobiles, or a reduction of societal dependence on alcohol.

14. My collection of soliloquies is heavily skewed. I have a large collection of such asides delivered by physicians, but very few from patients. Part of the reason for this is structural: I was simply "backstage" more frequently with the genetic counselors than I was with patients. But while structure is important, it does not explain everything. I found my more private moments with parents, listening to their stories, painful. As a result, I did not do everything I could and should have done to expand my corpus.

15. This paraphrase of T. S. Eliot's "The Hollow Men" is used here with some trepidation. For all I know, Eliot felt, like Auden, that thou shalt not "commit a social science."

port service, and as we shall see as well, that support is most routinely defined as factually correct medical information.

Fieldwork, then, provides a mirror for looking at who we are, as compared to who we would like to be. It provides us with soft data: observations, intuitions, and comments for rethinking some very hard questions about what it means to be a member of the society.

2

THE DOCTOR-PATIENT RELATIONSHIP IN CLINIC: ROUTINE WORK

So there I was, a worker in the field, a fellow professional invited to the conference table in order that the group might benefit from my specialized expertise, and much later a sociologist at a writing table. My analytic task, which I understood only very dimly, was to describe the doctor-patient relationship as it was understood in the context of the genetic counseling service of an elite, urban, academic pediatric center. My purpose, which shared vagueness with my task, was to show how one professional segment defined its mission, performed its core task, and understood its shared identity and fate (Bucher and Strauss 1961). I was lost in the field.

However, as an ethnographer, I had a set of tools to find my way. As a worker in the field, I would watch the genetic counselors at Nightingale work, and listen to their descriptions of that work. As a sociologist at a writing table, I use a number of shopfloor categories suggested by the workplace studies of Hughes and his students.[1]

1. The tagging of a body of work as "the program of Hughes and his students" needs both some bibliographic and some conceptual specificity. I have in mind the approach to work that is identified with the negotiated order of the workplace. As such, this body of work includes the studies of Ansèlm Strauss and his colleagues and students. *Negotiated order* is a broader rubric and for that reason perhaps a preferable way to identify the work at hand. Nonetheless, I prefer to identify the work more narrowly in terms of place, time, and people in order to give a historical sense of its production to provide a living rather than a purely literal tradition. Chapoulle (1987) provides a useful overview.

As a consequence, my description of genetic counselors' work at Nightingale has a specific style. The elements of that style are (1) first-hand observation as the fundamental method for understanding social life; (2) a dramaturgical interpretation of what happens in the various arenas in which genetic counselors work; (3) a structural differentiation of tasks into routines and emergencies as an integral feature of this occupational dramaturgy; (4) a concentrated focus on the neutralization of dirty work and everyday troubles within the context of routines and emergencies; and (5) a systematic attention in the analysis to the rough edges of professional practice: those places where professional and lay expectations about service are most problematic.[2]

This chapter discusses clinical work in the most routine scheduled form it took for genetic counselors: the weekly clinic. I will describe who came to genetic counselors and why. Then I will look at how counselors defined their counseling task. Next, I will examine how that task was then carried out in counseling sessions. Finally, I will look at how the counselors appraised their service.

Taken together, this chapter and the two that follow analyze the clinical work of genetic counselors as a recurrent source of everyday troubles and tasks, a set of normal, natural problems encountered at work. Our focus is on the solutions that the workgroup evolves to these everyday problems. While these troubles occurred

---

Representative work in this tradition includes the essays collected in Hughes (1971) and Becker (1970). Useful articles include Davis (1959), Roy (1952) and Gold (1952).

Within the sociology of medicine, Freidson (1970, 1976) and Goffman (1961a, Part 4) are useful overviews. Other representative work includes Stelling and Bucher (1972), Burkett and Knafl (1976), Sudnow (1967), Bosk (1979, 1980) Bosk and Frader (1990), Light (1980), Strauss, et al. (1964), and Strauss, et al. (1983), Guillemin and Holmstrom (1986).

2. While I am a student in this tradition, I am not a slavish adherent to it. In particular, there are two places where I have much trouble with this body of work. First, this work is marked by a rhetorical strategy that has as the ethnographer's main task to reverse the socially approved scales of vice and virtue used to describe occupations. While I engage in some of that kind of behavior, I do not take it as a main task. Second, the work in this tradition does not see the production of ethnographic texts as problematic. It is, however, difficult in contemporary ethnographic circles not to be impressed with some of the stylistic problems involved in the production of ethnographic texts as they have been discussed in Clifford and Marcus (1986), Clifford (1988), Rabinow and Sullivan (1979), Rabinow (1977), and Van Maanen (1988).

at multiple levels, three are most important in this description. First, there were clinical troubles as defined by the presenting complaints of patients. Patient's problems either revealed the depth of mastery which clinical geneticists had already obtained or, conversely, how little was known, how much remained to be done. The management of uncertainty, a recurrent theme in the sociology of medicine, was a routine feature of the work of genetic counselors.

Next, there were intragroup troubles. Here, the variety of approaches to the clinical troubles of patients exposed differences among the ways counselors defined their tasks. Simply put, as physicians, as professionals, the genetic counselors had an internalized obligation to do something for patients, to help them. On occasion, they disagreed as genetic counselors, as physicians, as professionals, and as people, as to what that help was. These disagreements appeared despite a shared and articulated commitment to both the value of patient autonomy and a nondirective, value-neutral ideology designed to promote it. As on most shopfloors, general principals were easier to agree on than cases. As a professional expert on medical services, as the witness to their recurring disagreements, and as a neutral field-worker, I tried never to arbitrate shopfloor disagreements unless explicitly asked to do so, and then I failed miserably.

Finally, there were intergroup troubles. In these cases, the presenting problems of patients and the suggested solutions for them pitted physicians against patients or physicians against physicians. There were cases where the proper standards of care were public issues. None of these cases were pleasant experiences for Nightingale Children's Center staff. Yet so long as Nightingale Children's claimed a place at the pinnacle of its specialization, such conflicts were unavoidable, however stressful they were for the workers in the institution. Without them, Nightingale would not have been on the cutting edge of pediatric care.

Genetic Counseling as Dirty Work

At Nightingale Children's Center, both diseases and medical specialties have regularly scheduled clinics. Chronic pediatric patients who suffered from conditions traceable to their genetic makeup or uterine development, problems such as spina bifida, cystic fibrosis, muscular dystrophy, hemophilia, and sickle-cell anemia, were treated by the appropriate subspecialty physicians in Nightingale's elaborate division of labor. The everyday clinical management of these conditions, even though they all may be understood as genetic problems, does not fall to members of the genetic counseling team. The genetic counselors did not provide routine treatment.

If genetic counselors do not treat patients with genetic disease at their clinic, who do they see, and what do they do for them? At the once-a-week, three-hour clinic that I observed, the genetic counselors met with either parents of "anomalous children" or prospective parents who either believed themselves to be, or were believed by others, most commonly their obstetricians, to be at risk for having a defective neonate. All those patients who requested visits to the clinic and who reported to the clinic fit one of three characterizations: (1) they had a known family history of a significant anomaly, (2) they were of "advanced maternal age," as categorized by the obstetrical standard of care, or (3) they had personal worries about exposure to pharmaceutical or environmental teratogens.

Couples, or more rarely individual women, received counseling from one of three physicians. *Bill Smith* who combined a residency in pediatrics with a fellowship in genetics. His offices were located at Nightingale Children's Center, and his responsibilities included organizing the group's clinical work. *Albert Samuels* was a "bench" researcher with offices and labs some blocks from Nightingale who had completed a residency in internal medicine and a fellowship in genetics. *Joseph Giordano* was a high-risk obstetrician whose clinical offices were located in an adjoining hospital. Counseling was sometimes provided by a nurse, *Mary O'Flynn,* who coordinated the amniocentesis testing for Giordano.[3] Very occasionally, a fourth

3. Here I have followed the conventions of ethnographic writing. Nightingale Children's Center is a made-up name for a real place. The names of the individuals who are characters in this ethnographic narrative are likewise aliases for real people. These aliases have been chosen with some attention to fidelity to the ethnicity of the real people involved. While providing specific details such as these compromises the confidentiality and anonymity that I as an ethnographer somewhat blithely promised my subjects, scrubbing my description of all local color robs the account of just those clues we need in order to understand why in this place at this time things were done one way rather than some other.

physician, either *Stuart Berger,* who was the group chief (Berger's occasional counseling was a result of his not taking on "new" clinic cases as he accepted responsibility for organizing Nightingale's Medical School's program in genetics research) or, after he left Nightingale Children's Center, his replacement as clinical chief, *Walter Palmer,* provided some counseling.

Just who could counsel patients was a hotly contested topic. The clinic coordinator, *Nancy Thomas,* who was a graduate of a two-year master's program in genetic counseling, and who agitated rather continually and forcefully for the opportunity to see patients, was consistently denied it. This denial rankled her, and she constantly referred to it as a major source of dissatisfaction with her job:

> I complain and complain about it [doing counseling]. And
> I've been told that I cannot because I am not a physician.
> It's a recurring frustration. It's one that I will have a
> discussion with Bill about every three or four months.
> Then I just get very, very angry, and it is that sort of thing.
> And it may mean I will eventually leave. I don't know that
> I can continually go on doing this forever . . . I don't feel
> I am capable of doing diagnostic work. I mean I certainly
> don't think that. I do think that there are certain situations
> in which I would be capable.

On a few occasions when she felt capable and confident, she incurred Bill Smith's ire by scheduling patients whose troubles she thought of as exceptionally mundane to see her on nonclinic days.

Nurse O'Flynn's access to patients was grudgingly allowed on only those occasions when Dr. Giordano was swamped and unable to manage his overload. Work contingencies necessitated this practice, which was not seen as violating group norms, since O'Flynn was merely "explaining a procedure," which was seen as different from "counseling patients." Moreover, even when O'Flynn did the "amnio-counseling," Giordano usually poked his head into the session and was introduced to the couple as the doctor-in-charge.

The fact that counseling patients was a jealously guarded physician prerogative at Nightingale reflects both the norms of the hospital and the aspirations of physicians who identified themselves as genetic counselors in the late 1970s and early 1980s. Genetic counseling is often carried out by other health-care professionals—most notably, social workers, nurses, psychotherapists, and those with graduate training in human genetics. Moreover, as recent growth in programs certifying genetic counselors indicates (Marks 1991), prenatal testing has become part of standard obstetrical care for designated categories of expectant mothers. The talking work of counseling has both moved down the division of labor to ancillary persons and out of the hospital, while obstetrician/gynecologists or perinatologists perform any necessary procedures. The necessary education and training for explaining prenatal tests is available to many, while many fewer are qualified to perform them.

When I conducted this research, the only therapeutic intervention that genetic counselors could recommend to patients was a second-trimester abortion. This has changed. A few centers now offer heroic *in utero* treatments to prevent selected birth defects.[4] Despite this miraculous change, genetic counseling can still be construed as a form of abortion counseling. Moreover, it is counseling for second-trimester abortions, which are more problematic than those in the first trimester, if for no other reason than the more compelling interest of the state in their regulation.[5]

Because of this, genetic counseling is central to the problem of abortion. The clinical activities of genetic counselors and the practice of selective abortion have been sources of controversy in public arenas. Luker's (1984) *Abortion and the Politics of Motherhood* locates the therapeutic abortions based on prenatal diagnosis as

4. As of this writing, the birth defects ameliorable *in utero* are all anatomical malformations. The interventions all involve fetal surgery, and have been discussed by Kolata (1990). There has yet to be an intervention for genetic conditions. However, given the time required for publication, this statement may no longer be true by the time this book appears. For a discussion, more generally, of the social, legal, and ethical problems presented by *in utero* interventions, see Bosk (1986).

5. *Roe v. Wade* balances the mother's right to privacy with the state's interest in protecting life by partitioning pregnancy into trimesters. The equation for balancing shifts with the trimester. As the pregnancy continues, the mother's interest wanes and the state's waxes. Underlying the logic of *Roe* is fetal viability. *Webster v. Missouri Health Services* places even greater emphasis than *Roe* on viability. With advances in fetal medicine, viability precedes the third trimester. Presumably, the interaction of technology and biology places a limit on when viability occurs, but the line keeps moving to earlier and earlier points in the pregnancy. With each shift of the line comes a diminution of the mother's reproductive rights.

the practice most hateful to the pro-life members of her sample and most benign to the pro-choice respondents.

> According to public opinion polls, such abortions [those intended to prevent the birth of a deformed child] are acceptable to more than four-fifths of the American public. However, . . . this one is the *least* ideologically acceptable for pro-life people. . . . abortions for fetal deformity cut to the deepest levels of pro-life feeling about "selective" abortion. Because the logic of abortion in this case depends upon a judgment that the embryo is "damaged" in one respect or another, it suggests to pro-life people the acceptance of the idea that humans can be ranked along some scale of perfection and that people who fall below a certain arbitrary standard can be excluded. . . . Already, for example, the movement is vigorously opposing amniocentesis, a diagnostic test performed on pregnant women to see if the embryo has any of a number of mental or physical handicaps. The present surgeon general of the United States, Everett Koop, an active pro-life supporter, has called amniocentesis exams "search and destroy missions," and the movement itself has labeled amniocentesis "selective genocide against the disabled." (P. 236)

For a number of reasons, it is peculiar that the physicians of Nightingale guard the privilege of seeing those referred for counseling, whom they always call *patients* and never *clients*. After all, abortion counseling qualifies as social dirty work, and such work is normally shunned by physicians. Moreover, in this case the work is politically controversial. We know from Imber's (1986) work that performing abortions can make physicians pariahs in the local community. Why are these tertiary-care physicians different? Why is it that a group of physicians both wanted and were able to claim successfully a task normally avoided? Moreover, how is second-trimester abortion, which in public arenas is so problematic, managed in the context of the doctor-patient relationship so that it is a routine and private, albeit difficult, enterprise?

The genetic counselors were able to insulate themselves from the public debate over abortion because of the political epidemiology of their practice. Clinic users were of two types: (1) childless couples or women who had deferred child-rearing, and (2) families who had had an affected child. Their appearance at Nightingale made it more likely that they had private health insurance. The abortion debate has been unfolding along a different line than that of the propriety of "selective abortion." Rather, the line of attack on women's reproductive rights has been the use of public funds to perform abortion services. Clinics providing more basic reproductive counseling to the poor and uninsured have not been able to distance themselves from the public debate about abortion. Genetic counselors not only distance themselves, but the very techniques that are being developed in the labs hold the promise that one day genuine therapies may be dispensed and the conditions that give rise to "selective abortions" remedied. Although they recognized its limitations and were aware of the difficulties involved in measuring it, the genetic counselors at Nightingale believed that they had some help to dispense. They could provide diagnostic information that would allow patients to make their own choices, something that all the genetic counselors agreed was part of the patient's natural right. Their expert neutrality could clarify the situation for the patient. As physicians, the genetic counselors were in a peculiar situation. They had an obligation to act, to help the patient; but to satisfy this obligation, they had to refrain from taking charge of decision making. They had to act, but not decisively. In clinic, the genetic counselor provides information that informs reproductive decision making or that medically labels the severely damaged.

Routine Problems and Normal Risks

One key for understanding how the genetic counselors define expert neutrality is to look at the information they provide to patients and what issues are kept out of a counseling session. Focusing on what counselors say during counseling allows us to understand how they define their task, how they understand their work, and how they place boundaries around their professional responsibilities. This is easy to do, for genetic counseling sessions are goal-oriented. For those who bring in a child with anomalies, genetic counselors seek to provide a diagnosis, to say conclusively whether the particular pattern of birth anomalies is attributable to a genetic syndrome with a known recurrence risk. They seek to inform all prospective parents of the conditions for which their children are at risk, to provide the conditional probabilities that those risks will materialize, and to describe any existing methods of prenatal diagnosis, as well as the time frame for making a decision to abort or not in case of a positive diagnosis.

The genetic counselors' expert neutrality and nondirective style further distance them from the public and politically problematic dimensions of second-trimester abortion. They simply calculate the probabilities for pregnancy outcomes and recite the conditional probabilities to those who have sought their advice. The choice among these alternatives is felt to be the couple's private business. In general, the only follow-up to the single informational session provided by a clinic visit is a letter which summarizes the discussion. It is not that counselors do not care what couples do; rather, they are careful not to be too intrusive in the decision-making process.

Despite their commitment to nondirective, neutral, information-based counseling, invariably the counselors shape the way that information is presented to prospective parents in ways that are geared to influence private risk assessment and decision making. This arises from the way the risk statements that genetic counselors use to frame alternatives are constructed. First, all risk statements are comparative. One goal of counseling is to have prospective parents understand their own risks in relation to those of the normal population. The normal population risk for having a child with a birth defect which the counselors quote to their clients is 3 percent.[6] This is a figure which surprises most clients who assume that birth is less risky than that.

On the one hand, the very fact that risks can be expressed in numeric form allows counselors, if they choose, to merely pass information on to clients in an objective fashion; for example, "The

---

6. Gusfield's (1981) discussion of why we find scientific numbers compelling and how they can be misleading applies to this number as well. For a general discussion of the problems with a scientific number and the popular media discourse about cancer risks, see Hilgartner (1990).

normal population risk is 3 percent. Your risk is 6 percent." Such precise statements underscore the counselor's objectivity, neutrality, and commitment to the scientific data. Such risk statements without elaboration are rare. On the other hand, the numeric form of risk statements allows counselors to make statements about risk in ways that will imply what a reasonable and responsible person will do with the information. For example, consider the difference between the following statements, each of which is correct: "Your risk is 3 percent greater than that of the general population" and "Your risk is double that of the general population." Risk statements of the latter form are more common than bare, unelaborated numbers, despite the counselors' commitment to not intruding on the privacy of patient decision making. Risk statements by counselors were framed so that patients could either appreciate the seriousness or the triviality of the problem.

How much higher the specific risks are than this general 3 percent estimate is one of two factors that counselors use in constructing the seriousness of the "story"[7] that they tell patients. The other factor is the nature of the defects for which the couple is at risk. As a rule, the most serious defects involve retardation or death in the first two years of life. The kinds of abnormalities that involve merely those deviations from normal appearances that Goffman (1961b) associated with stigma or spoiled identity are viewed less seriously.

> Bill Smith is counseling a couple whose daughter was born with a seriously deformed right hand: the thumb is normally developed, the fifth finger is curved in and not fully developed, the second finger is present, the third and fourth fingers are absent. Bill has consulted with a radiologist and the teratologist associated with the group. They have advised him that this is an isolated anomaly; it is neither lobster claw nor Crouzon's syndrome, each of which has a specific recurrence risk.
>
> In meeting with the parents, Bill assures them that, "Your baby's problems are not associated with anything

---

7. Quotation marks here are meant to signify that this term is the work argot among counselors and not a trendy theoretical contrivance signaling my interest in the primacy of narrative in the social construction of reality.

else. . . . It [the hand] is a totally isolated finding—you
have a totally normal, healthy baby. . . . The real
important thing for you to remember is that you have a
normal baby, as long as everybody treats her as normal.
She checks out normal on our charts. There are a lot of
things that happen to an embryo, and it's like an
orchestra, and when you think about it, it is amazing that
all the things go right. But the important thing to
remember is that her children and your children, your
future children that is, will all be normal."

But how is a baby with that hand normal? Surely the hand will have
some impact on this child's life, will restrict the range of activities in
which she can take part. And how to get everyone to treat her as
normal when she has the kind of visible defect that makes passing
impossible, is hard to disattend in interaction, and spoils identity
(Goffman 1961b)? Bill is able to give the parents the counsel he
does because, in general, the counselors use a version of the social
capacity theory of personhood. The critical capacity for counselors
is, as it is for other physicians, normal intelligence or cognitive
functioning (Crane 1976). At the same time, Bill recognizes the im-
possibility of his own counsel. In the postclinic conference, he
states that he thinks the baby will always be known as "the one with
the hand."

Expert Explanations

However surprising the fact that genetic counseling is something
done almost exclusively by physicians at Nightingale Children's
Center, the provision of this service by these professionals has important consequences for its definition and delivery, not the least of
which is that it frames the couple's or woman's previously personal
and private existential dilemma ("What to do?") in the context of a
medical relationship with its own rules for action.

The provision of this service by physicians also shapes its con-
tents. The genetic counselors emphasize the scientific/technical
side of the data they present to parents. A point of pride with the
genetics team is their thoroughness:

I know that by the time that somebody gets here, it's as
close to the truth as it's going to be. I mean I feel
confident in that . . . in terms of technical ability, in terms
of laboratory work. When something gets done, I feel that
it's been done to its best, that there are no stones
unturned.

This thoroughness and technical proficiency are marked in multiple ways. In the weekly preclinic conference, a goodly amount of
discussion about what to tell patients centers around reports in the
literature. Little attention is paid to who the patients are, their social
circumstances, level of education, amount of distress, and so on.
Each genetic condition has its own "complete story," that needs to
be told and is independent of the patient being counseled.

For the most exotic conditions, counselors initiate phone contacts with "big names" at other institutions to make certain that no
recent developments in chromosome-banding and staining which
have implications for *in utero* diagnosis have escaped their attention. A number of encyclopedias of birth anomalies are kept on
hand during clinic, so that findings from patient exams can be cor-
related with reported clinical data. The emphasis in genetic counseling is quite clearly on genetics as a science, rather than on counseling as a relational process.

During sessions with parents, counselors use a number of devices to dramatize either that they have an explanation for a child's
aberrant development or that they can assign a specific risk to a
pregnancy. When a problem was chromosomal, the counselors always displayed the photographic karyotype.

Bill Smith is counseling a couple who have come in for
an explanation of the problems of their severely
retarded, five-year-old daughter, who has little language
and is just beginning toilet training. He pulls out of the
chart he is holding a cardboard-mounted karyotype,
passes it to the parents, and begins to talk: "We did a
number of complicated chromosomal tests; we think we
know what her problem is. If you'll look at this, you'll see
this is a picture of chromosomes. And you'll see here,
where this arrow is, this chromosome is longer than the

one next to it. We think this extra piece which is on the
9th chromosome is the cause of all her problems. And we
think that's why she has the problems that she does, why
she has this delay, and why she's slow. We took your
chromosomes. . . . and we think it's a spontaneous
mutation that occurred in your child for reasons that we
don't know."

Bill Smith is meeting with the Chilmarks, a couple
whose child is in the neonatal intensive care unit. Bill
begins the discussion: "I think we have as much of an
answer as we are ever going to get. Your baby has an extra
piece of chromosomal material. Look at the karyotype we
did of your baby. [Here he passes the picture to the
parents.] The 6 is here; part of it seems to be missing, but
it's really here at the bottom of this chromosome [he
points to 18]. On banding, we see that most of the 6 is
here. The top is equivalent to 18, but the 18 is trisomic;
that means there are three pieces of it.

This routine display of photographs and the expert decoding of
them is also a regular feature of the counseling for couples who
come in for advanced maternal age. Ultrasound photographs and
karyotypes are shown to parents to help aid their understanding of
how prenatal diagnosis works. They are evidence of the real problem.

Of course, such photographic displays can only be a feature of
chromosomal disorders. Other types of disorders call for different
dramatizations of scientific expertise and different representations
of biological processes. For recessive disorders, the counselors
draw Mendelian diagrams on pieces of paper for prospective parents to give them a better understanding of their reproductive risks.
When counselors cannot display the problem in a photograph or
display recurrence risks in a diagram, they deliver to parents long
didactic lectures on specific genetic disorders.

Albert Samuels is counseling the Menemshas, a couple
who have a child with an antibody deficiency. He begins

the session: "What I have to tell you today is very complicated—there's no clear answer to why Teddy has his antibody deficiency. You're going to have to know an awful lot about genetics to follow what I say. We have to assume it's a genetics problem. Now there are many problems with antibody deficiencies that are inherited. . . . Now let's start at the beginning. Genes come in pairs, and there are thousands of them on chromosomes. Now when an egg fertilizes a sperm, each takes one of the chromosomes, so there's a 50-50 chance of any member of a gene pair being inherited from a mother or a father. Now in these antibody disorders, there are three modes of inheritance. They can either be sex-linked, recessive, or a new mutation." Samuels then goes on to explain each of these and their associated recurrence risk.

The counselor's explanation of genetic disease described the cause to parents in impersonal, distant, abstract, technical terms: "this part of the photograph where the arrow is" or "we all have bad genes. It's just an event, a random and tragic accident that these genes get passed on in just the right order to produce conditions like Kevin has . . ." To soften the blow of having a child born with significant birth defects, the genetic counselors speak of normal birth as a symphonic miracle. Yet in translating their technical understanding of why this miracle fails to occur, the genetic counselors are forced into an everyday language that equates the miraculous to mundane matters such as proper switching and correct copying. Problems of the central nervous system, for example, always involve analogies to zippers functioning properly and are represented by folding sheets of paper into tubes.

Their relentless focus on the scientific, technical side of patient problems permits counselors to dramatize their expertise and also to avoid engaging a raft of emotional issues raised by the presence of genetic disease. In fact, the genetic counselors often find managing this emotional work outside their domain of expertise as physicians. So much is this the case that this work is "turfed" by the counselors to the genetic associate, who, despite the general prohibition against her seeing patients, is allowed to meet with them for this "nonspecialized" part of the counseling task.

> I remember feeling somewhat confused the first time that
> Bill said to me, "Go in and mop up." I mean I just didn't
> know what that meant when I first started here. I have
> since learned that what it means is to just sit and let
> people talk. But they do not want to do that with another
> person.

Not only was the genetic associate used this way, but I was often assigned to observe those cases that the genetic counselors assumed would have the heaviest emotional overtones. Often I was asked to interview these patients following their sessions. As a researcher, I was thus also co-opted into providing "mop-up" services as well.

Counselors attempted to avoid the most problematic aspects of their work by confining their task to scientific information and impersonal risk statements. Such a task definition, they felt, was the only way possible to allow patients to make their own decisions—it was the only way to preserve patient autonomy in the highly charged area of reproductive decision making. Nonetheless, counselors routinely delivered risk statements in ways that undercut the formal commitment to nondirective counseling.

For example, the bulk of the patients who were offered prenatal diagnosis had as their presenting problem advanced maternal age.[8] In these cases, the genetic counselors spoke of amniocentesis as a device for reducing parental anxiety and providing reassurance:

> Giordano is counseling a couple who have recently lost a
> child. The mother is forty, and Giordano begins to
> explain amniocentesis to her: "The chances are overall 2–

8. Not surprisingly, it turns out that advanced maternal age is somewhat elastic. At the beginning of my field research, women forty years old or older were considered to be "of advanced maternal age." However, a number of studies documenting the safety and efficacy of amniocentesis, as well as a spate of lawsuits brought for "wrongful birth" by couples who had children with birth defects diagnosable *in utero,* reduced the age of mothers for whom the procedure was recommended form forty to thirty-five.

3 percent of having a kid with a birth defect. But the
chances of having a child with Down's increases with age.
Look (Giordano takes a piece of paper and draws a
graph), if this is the age of mothers and this is the chance
of having a kid with Down's, you can see the following:
For a 20-year-old, the chance of having a baby with
Down's is 1 in 1500, and it stays like that till about age 29,
when it begins to climb. It gradually climbs until about
35. Then it really goes up, so that the chances between 35
and 40 of having a child with Down's syndrome are
between 1 and 250. With the test, we can bring your odds
back to those of a 20 year old."

When discussing amniocentesis, counselors often claimed the procedure brought the risk of having an affected child down to "below"
the normal population risk since many conditions the normal population risk included were screened for by the procedure.

In general, when a prenatal screening mechanism existed for a
condition, it was offered to parents with the same enthusiasm that
amniocentesis was offered to women of advanced maternal age.
Couples were reassured that their chances of having a perfect baby
were higher than average. Genetic counselors neutralized whatever stigma adhered to their work as "abortion counselors" by re-
minding themselves and others that (1) a significant number of
couples who would not have borne children without the services
provided at the counseling center did so, and that (2) patients were
never coerced; they remained free to make their own choices.

The Rough Edge of Professional Practice

The counselors' task was relatively unproblematic when they could
tell patients "good stories," which contained either a firm diagnostic label or the existence of a prenatal test or both. In these situations, the counselors passed their information to the patients and
passed as well a sense that whatever decision a couple made was a
private one. From the counselors' perspective, these stories
worked for two reasons: they provided a clear and coherent account of what happened, and they provided a strategy for avoiding
the occurrence of a dreaded condition.

Problems developed when a particular condition could not be diagnosed, when there was no appropriate prenatal test, or where parents at risk appeared unwilling to utilize available tests. Each of these situations presented a different facet of the "rough edge" of professional practice.

When a particular condition can not be diagnosed, or when no prenatal diagnosis exists, genetics counselors face the limits of their craft; they are reminded of the clinical impotence that Parsons (1951) characterizes as a fundamental existential ground of the physician's role. Simply put, the very cognitive mastery that clinicians possess exposes them to the futility of intervention. This impotence often disappoints parents who are looking for solutions to very pressing problems.

When a diagnosis cannot be made, the genetic counselors try to counter parental disappointment by making the best of a bad situation. They reassure parents that the failure to come up with a firm diagnosis will in the future rebound to a child's benefit, since the child will be treated as an individual and not as a person with a syndrome.

> We are in the preclinic conference. Samuels is presenting a patient who is coming in for counseling at this week's clinic. The patient is a sixteen-year-old male who presented at a local hospital with lower back pain, headaches, and nasal congestion. He also had short incurved fingers, and these were the reason that the physicians had referred him to the genetics group. Samuels said that he was presenting the case to find out if there was anything that the group wanted to do. How extensively should the patient be worked up? Samuels suggested that the patient be extensively worked up. There were two components to his urging. First, there was the sheer scientific interest, the possibility of discovering a new syndrome or an exotic variant of some documented one, Second, he suggested a diagnosis might reduce anxiety by pointing to a cause for the patient's problems.
>
> Berger objects to Samuels's reasoning. He claims that

the best thing to do in this case would be nothing at all, that there was no reason to pin a genetics label on the patient. He said the patient should be treated as a normal sixteen-year-old who had abdominal pains and headaches, all suggestive of growing pains, and leave it at that.

The group agrees to Berger's and not Samuel's plan for treatment after only cursory discussion in which there is no support for an extensive work-up.

Berger is reporting in the postclinic conference on a child that he saw that afternoon. He reported that he was able to get a great history because the mother is a nutritionist, and the father works as an engineer. The child was brought in for diagnosis because of a big head and "an unusual appearance that seems to be a family trait." The child has been slow to gain weight and slow to reach developmental milestones. He has had a number of febrile illnesses with seizures. The parents are anxious to have a reason and a name for his problems. He has been worked up at three other renowned pediatric centers for his problems. All three failed to come up with a diagnosis. Berger counseled the parents that they were better off this way, because the child would be treated as an individual and not a syndrome. Although the family was "super-anxious and guilty," Berger discouraged any work-up of their child.

The restraint counselors display when it comes to applying labels fits well with their desire to preserve patient autonomy and privacy; by not labeling patients, counselors preserve the claims of those patients to normal treatment. As we shall see shortly, preserving privacy is not without its costs.[9]

9. This restraint is also not without some interest to medical sociologists, who have suggested that medical professionals are somewhat imperialistic about label-ing. We have, to date, no analyses of medical reluctance to label. Rather, we have extensive discussions of overreaching when it comes to labeling. By not beginning to pay attention to professionals' reluctance to label, we are overlooking one of the

Work with patients who have considerable anxiety about the risk of a pregnancy, but for whom no prenatal test exists also exposes a rough edge of genetic counseling. When I was in the field, the classic example of this was Huntington's chorea (Woody Guthrie's disease), a fatal, degenerative neuromuscular disorder of long duration.[10] Huntington's chorea is an autosomal dominant disorder. This means that the child of an affected individual has a 50 percent probability of inheriting the condition and subsequently passing it on to his or her own children. At the time of this research, no test for carrier status existed.[11] Since the disease does not manifest itself until the late thirties or early forties, the children of an affected parent faced a complex set of personal anxieties about themselves and very difficult decisions about reproductive decision making.

> I am in a counseling session with Samuels. A husband
> and wife have come in with the wife's mother for
> counseling. The wife's father had Huntington's. At the
> beginning of the session, the wife's mother was quite
> talkative. Her talk reflected that she was quite guilty about
> having had two children with an affected spouse. She
> kept repeating that "back then" no one knew anything
> about Huntington's chorea, that had she known she might

---

direct effects of the widespread dispersion of labeling theories of deviance. We are overlooking one of the domains in which sociological work has had an impact on professional practice.

10. It is interesting that the other disease known to the public by a celebrity eponym, Lou Gerhig's disease, or amyotrophic muscular sclerosis, is a degenerative neuromuscular disorder as well. It is also interesting that celebrities have played a role not only by bringing the disease to public attention but also by organizing a secondary network of patient advocacy and support groups, research foundations, fundraising, and public-interest associations.

The secondary organization around specific disease labels or categories is an interesting topic for research, but one that falls outside the scope of this inquiry.

11. A test now exists for carrier status. Individuals who seek the test must also agree to undergo psychological evaluation beforehand to determine if they can cope with positive test results, and counseling afterward to help them cope with the results. The fact that Huntington's testing has changed has not made the counseling questions posed by the disease any easier. The basic problems posed by the absence of a prenatal test for a specific condition has been resolved for this condition, but not for others.

have had second thoughts about having her children.[12]
She mentioned as well that the father's sister is at present
hospitalized with the condition and that the wife's
brother has two children.

After Samuels took a detailed clinical history of the
disease's progression in the two family members affected,
both the husband and wife asked repeatedly if a test
existed for seeing if the wife was affected or if a child
would be affected. Each time they asked, Samuels told
them that unfortunately the answer was no.

The couple then asked what people in their situation
do. Samuels told them first that he did not know what
people in their situation did. He then told them that what
other people did was not necessarily a relevant
consideration for them. He stressed that they were
unique individuals with their own set of values.

The couple then engaged Samuels in the likelihood of
testing in the near future. Samuels was unwilling to
speculate how long it would be before testing was
available.

The couple asked again what other people did in their
position. Samuels again replied that he did not know. He
suggested that if the couple was really curious, they use
the Huntington's Chorea Foundation to speak to others
who had faced the decision themselves.

Samuel's response to patient uncertainty about reproductive decision making is characteristic of the counselors as a group.

The commitment to a nondirective style leads counselors to respond to the question, "What should we do?" with a didactic lecture
about how only the couple can know what is right for them, and to

12. Such talk by mothers in front of their hearing children was not uncommon
and not only for Huntington's. Genetic counselors with another agenda did not respond to this talk. I always assumed that the mothers who talked this way in front of
strangers had expressed similar sentiments to their children at home, that they presented familiar familial laments, and that they had been worked through. I never
explored the bearing of such laments on offspring's sense of identity, esteem, or
security.

respond to the follow-up question, "What do others in our situation do?" by dismissing the relevance of the question because each individual couple is in its own unique situation. The question, "What should we do?" is raised most frequently in those cases where no prenatal testing occurs and where risk is high.[13] Counselors do not use the question to explore what the parents' values are or what they think they should do. Counselors invite a couple to talk about their decision, but not with them. It is a personal issue, a familial issue, a communal one, but not a question for this professional relationship. Rather, they use the question to highlight the couple's privacy and autonomy, and they point them toward other resources, including advocacy and support groups.

Occasionally, presenting couples with clear directives was a source of tension for the genetic counselors. This was especially so when members of the group disagreed with one another about those clear directives.

> Giordano is counseling the Goldbergs, a couple who
> recently had an infant with multiple anomalies who died.
> He started the session by saying, "I think that the news we
> have for you is good. We had the embryologist review the
> records of your child, and he thinks that the multiple
> malformations were an accident, one of those things that
> just happen in a pregnancy. He thinks that you are people
> who face the normal population risk of a birth defect and
> also, the normal population chance of having a normal
> child."
>
> The Goldbergs smiled at this, sat back and relaxed in
> their chairs, and then hunched forward. After a long
> pause, Giordano asked, "Do you have any questions?"
>
> Mrs. Goldberg responded immediately: "Yes, what
> does it mean the embryologist reviewed the file? What
> did he do?"
>
> Giordano answered, "Certain birth defects are
> accidental in that they occur at just one moment in the

13. *High risk* is of course a vague term. But the conditions that most frequently fit this description are those with the following known modes of transmission: autosomal dominant—50 percent inheritance; autosomal recessive—25 percent inheritance; X-linked recessive disorders—these affect only males, but not all males.

pregnancy. They are not inborn errors in the genetic code. Our assumption is that if the birth defect is due to a chromosomal or genetic anomaly, which is true in only a very limited number of conditions, then the birth defect will express itself during the entire pregnancy, during each stage of the pregnancy, since it was planned there from the beginning, since it's part of the genetic package and makeup of the fetus. However, certain things are accidental in the sense that the same accident, the same event, is not likely to occur at the same time in another pregnancy. Now, when the embryologist reviewed the file, he dated the number of defects in your child and found that they all occurred at roughly the same time in the pregnancy. This made him think that it was a chance event and that it was unlikely to happen again."

Mrs. Goldberg asked, "Is there any reason why this accident occurred?"

Giordano said, "There are any number of things that could happen, but it is really impossible to pinpoint a single cause. It is clear, however, that there is nothing you did in the pregnancy that would have caused this to happen. There are a lot of people who feel guilty after a child is born, and they say things like, 'Well, if I hadn't been angry, or if I hadn't gone to the party, or if I hadn't caught a cold . . .' Now we know that there are only a certain number of events for which that is true, like measles. And we know that none of these events happened for you. Therefore, we feel relatively safe saying nothing that you did could have changed the outcome one bit. So, I guess I'd say to you, go ahead and plan to have another child, just don't worry anymore than you have to that the child will be normal. Now you'll probably worry a little bit more than most people because you had this unfortunate experience. What we're telling you is that this experience should have no relationship to future pregnancies."

After a bit more questioning, the Goldbergs left the session all smiles.

Giordano's certainty in reassuring the Goldbergs was striking. He did not, as is usually the case, stress that there was no guarantee of a healthy child. He did not, as is usually the case, double the normal population risk based on their prior unhappy outcome.

The lack of hedging which marks most discourse between physicians and patients was quite striking and did not prepare me for what was soon to follow.

> At the clinic conference, Giordano was presenting the case of the Goldbergs. Berger listened to Giordano's description and then asked, "Joe, is there any evidence that merely because something happens at a single point in embryo genesis that it is not a genetic disease?"
>
> Giordano answered, "No, and frankly I feel a little uncomfortable about the clinical counseling that we're doing based upon this viewpoint, since things that appear different can be a single phenomenon, and because there is such a narrow time frame involved in the dating anyway, that it's likely that many things connected with a single cause could occur at the same time."
>
> Berger stated that he too was skeptical of this approach and began to worry when they used unconfirmed theories as clinical guidelines.

Until Berger asked his question, it was not apparent that any uncertainty existed at all. It was as if the genetic counselors were acting in that state that Matza (1964) describes as "pluralistic ignorance," each group member keeping his questions, doubts, and hesitancies private, lest voicing them prove the group member to lack the courage of his or her convictions. Nonetheless, Berger's question created considerable apprehension that the genetic counselors were acting inappropriately by being so reassuring. The acknowledgment of uncertainty dissolved the group consensus and created great distrust of the clear directive "not to worry" given to the patients.

On other occasions as well, counselors felt that the clear directives given patients were wrong, and considerable conflict and anxiety was created in the group. Such open conflict was rare, but it did occur.

The Mulroneys are coming in for genetic counseling. They have a child with tuberous sclerosis. Mr. and Mrs. Mulroney have been worked up for signs of the condition in its mildest form. Mr. Mulroney was found to have a hypopigmented, ash-leaf macule on his upper left arm, which was visible under a Woods lamp. Despite this finding, Berger intends to counsel the Mulroneys that they have no increased risk for tuberous sclerosis.

The rest of the group is quite upset. During the preclinic conference, they argued with Berger that the presence of the white spot could not be chalked up to chance. Berger disagreed. He maintained that no one knew what percentage of people in the general population had white spots, and it might be a quite common finding. As the group pressed the point, Berger got visibly angry and said that he wanted to hear no more about it.

Bill left the conference quite agitated. He claimed that the group needed Berger's expertise and couldn't tolerate his falling apart over a patient and not seeing what was in front of his nose. He vowed to spend the rest of the week softening Berger up. Whatever happened, he said, there was no way that he was going to allow him to counsel these patients that they had no increased recurrence risk.

Bill immediately did a literature review on hypopigmented ash-leaf macules. He uncovered a study done in France which surveyed 9,000 families, of which only 60 had white spots. He interpreted this data to mean that (1) the presence of white spots was sufficiently rare that one could not say with certainty that they were not significant and that (2) the presence of white spots in more than one family member, given their overall low incidence, certainly had to be interpreted as evidence that the father was possibly a carrier of the disease.

Before clinic, Bill and Giordano went to see Berger. Bill displayed the results of his literature review. Berger dismissed them as showing nothing more than the presence of white spots means there are white spots in some families. Giordano began to talk about what he called "the bias of ascertainment." By this, he meant that, originally, only the most severe expressions of disorder were thought to represent autosomal dominant disorders and, as a result, most autosomal dominant disorders were thought to be new mutations in families without affected individuals. Increasingly, members of the genetics group are finding subclinical manifestations of the disease in other family members. Berger was impatient with this argument as well. He said that there were problems enough in clinical genetics without making up new genetic diseases and new categories of who was going to inherit a disease and who not.

Bill was now really upset. He asked me to observe Berger with the Mulroneys so I could "tell them all what really happened in the session."

During the session, Berger reported to the Mulroneys that as far as he was concerned there was nothing in their work-ups to indicate that either of the parents carried the gene for tuberous sclerosis; that, as far as he was concerned, their affected child was just one of those things, a random event. Berger went so far as to say that if they had a second child with tuberous sclerosis, they would be written up in medical textbooks. Then he asked, rhetorically, "How often do people get written up in medical textbooks?"

The week after this session, Mrs. Mulroney, trying to get in touch with Berger, who was out of town, reached Bill by phone. She reported that she had found a white spot on the chest wall of her other child, previously thought to be unaffected. Bill refused to tell her anything save she should speak to Berger.

The group, in this case, is in conflict with its leader. It tries all the modes known to subordinates to get the leader to budge: the gentle question, the extensive literature review, the personal conference. Yet, when all these fail, they find themselves impotent to change a counseling strategy which they think verges on error. The uncertainties built into the structure of what is known, combined with differences among group members in assessing risk, all contribute here to making this rough edge all the more jagged. In this case, the problem was confounded because the information that there was no risk of recurrence risk was disputed. If risks are falsely assessed, the genetic counseling undermines the rational choice and patient autonomy the service was intended to promote.

Couples to whom they could not provide clear directives posed one type of problem to genetic counselors; couples to whom they provided clear directives which were in dispute posed another. Couples who were provided with clear directives but who chose to ignore them posed a third problem. In these cases the counselors were torn between their commitment to nonjudgmental, nonintrusive information-giving and their sense of appropriate behavior.

> I was with Samuels in a counseling session with parents who had just lost a child to Werdnig-Hoffman's disease. Samuels had explained that the condition was always lethal, that the couple had a one-in-four recurrence risk, and that no prenatal diagnosis existed.
>
> Samuels was closing the session and asked the couple how they felt about all the information that they had heard thus far. The husband responded, "I guess we'll just go home and flip a coin."
>
> Samuels responded very negatively to this. He stressed that it was a very serious decision because of the emotional, financial, and social consequences for the family. He repeated that artificial insemination was an option for this family. I got the impression that he was quite distressed that they would consider another pregnancy.

What is striking here is that even though Samuels disagrees with this couple's appreciation of the seriousness of the problem and with their approach to it, he is not able to make his disagreement explicit. Rather, he merely repeats to them information he had previously communicated about the magnitude of the problem and possible solutions for it.

When couples act in ways that the counselors find inexplicable or indefensible, the counselors remind themselves of their mandate to communicate information to patients and not to make difficult choices for them.

It is a Friday afternoon at postclinic conference. Bill Smith is providing some follow-up on the Meullers, a couple who had recently been in for counseling. Bill explains that the Meullers are a couple who have recently had a child with Von Recklinghausen's disease. Mr. Meuller has four café au lait spots (a marker of this dominant condition in its less serious manifestations). He has been seen by a number of physicians, two of whom thought the spots meant that he carried the gene. Bill then asked Giordano to continue. He first described the counseling session he had had with them and then described a conversation with the Meuller's pediatrician. The pediatrician knew how much Mrs. Meuller did not want an abortion and was angry at the clinic for assigning carrier status to Mr. Meuller without a skin biopsy.

Giordano continued: "To make a long story short, Mr. and Mrs. Meuller went shopping for a dermatologist who said that the spots did not definitely mean that he carried the gene. Mrs. Meuller called today to say that she was going to keep the pregnancy."

Giordano, Smith and Samuels are all distressed that Mrs. Meuller is going to carry this pregnancy to term. They all believe that there is at least a 50 percent chance that the infant will have the disease (although the seriousness of expression ranges from Mr. Meuller's café au lait spots to the features of the Elephant Man).

Giordano sums up with an expression of helplessness. Having sized up his options, he says, "The only thing I can accomplish if I intervene is harm."

Bill Smith says, "I want to sum up for your benefit, Bosk. This is a couple who have chosen to minimize and deny the risk, who are bound and determined to keep the pregnancy. This is a different situation than the

Allegra's (other clinic patients), who are trying to decide
whether or not to take the risk. These people (the
Meullers), are ignoring it entirely. There are three
different situations to worry about. Cases where parents
accept a very high risk, cases where they deny there is any
risk at all, and cases where they can't get the meaning of
the risk clear in their own minds."

Genetic counselors worry when patients act in ways that appear
unreasonable to them. They worry, but they do not exert much
pressure beyond the conversational give-and-take of the single
counseling session. For example, they do not suggest follow-up
sessions for patients who clearly ignore, deny, or do not understand serious risk. It is somewhat hard to discriminate what part of
this behavior is determined by a professional ideology that en-
codes standards of proper practice and what part by a concern for
patient finances. Rather, the counselors remind themselves that
"we do not give our patients their genes, and we don't plan their
pregnancies."

The genetic counselors' distress when patients do not appear
ready to heed their advice or do not appear to understand it is often
expressed in the "black" humor that characterizes medical settings
more generally.

In the postclinic conference, Bill Smith is talking about
the first case he had today, a sixteen-year-old who had a
child with Cornelia de Lange syndrome. Bill said that he
couldn't get through to her—this was a girl with very
long bangs, and when she put her head down, you had
nothing to talk to, you couldn't see any part of her face.
Bill said that the mother wanted things in black-and-white
terms, that she wanted them simple, that all she really
understood was that she'd had a baby and now she didn't
get to take the baby home, and that she was very upset
about that. Bill said that he never felt that he got through
to the mother how it was a terrible disease, how the
infant was severely retarded, and how the infant was
going to die soon. All the mother could understand,

according to Bill, was that she had a baby and she didn't
take a baby home.

On hearing this, Al Samuels said, "That's the best
argument I've heard all day for tubal ligation."

To this, Giordano responded, "Al's got about two or
three years left of genetic counseling before we have to
put him in a closet." The group began to laugh, and then
Giordano added, "Al's already at the point where he's
ready to clone just the good people." The laughter grew
louder.

The joke here for the group is on Samuels for his frustration with
the nondirective role—a frustration shared by all the members of
the group. The joke is then re-keyed. This time Giordano's Promethean vision of a world where cloning is technically possible and
morally acceptable to genetic counselors as frustrated as Samuels is
seen for the modest Swiftian proposal that it is. Similar jokes were
made whenever parents did not seem to appreciate the seriousness
of their children's problems or their own reproductive risks. Such
jokes formed a running commentary about the difficulties of providing, defining, and delivering a valuable professional service.

The Patient's Side of the Rough Edge

The rough edge of everyday practice for genetic counselors grows
out of those situations where available technology fails to provide
patients with a screening test or where patients fail to hear correctly
the statements made about risk. Not surprisingly, the rough edge is
somewhat different for patients. To borrow from Merton (1957), if
genetic counselors are cosmopolitan when understanding genetic
disease, patients are locals. In everyday terms this means that genetic counselors' explanations are framed in universal terms. They
are valid not just for the current couple receiving counseling, but
for all patients in this disease category. Explanations are focused on
abstract, impersonal, biological processes. Conversely, patient understandings are very specific and personal. They are fashioned out
of highly situated understandings for this particular pregnancy, this
particular family, this particular person. Unlike the genetic coun-

selors, patients focus on the concrete. To borrow again, this time from Lévi-Strauss (1966), genetic counselors aspire to act in idealized models of scientific action; patients are like *bricoleurs:* they take what they can and fashion out of it something that works, something that sustains understanding.

For many patients, the counselor's best case—a screening test with an abortion for a positive diagnosis—is problematic. Counselors assume that voluntarily showing up for clinic means that patients are at least willing to hear this alternative. In any case, as counselors carry out their work, their troubles end where the patient's begin. For one thing, the risk figures that the genetic counselors disclose, like all risk figures that physicians disclose to patients, are risk figures for a population. A 3-percent, or 25-percent, or 50-percent risk is, in any case, a theoretic risk. For the couple making a decision, this theoretic figure is of somewhat limited utility. It can serve as a guide to decision making. Nonetheless, for them, the risk will materialize or it will not. In any given case, the *a posteriori* odds are 0 or 100 percent. Understanding the difference between theoretic risk and materialized event makes clear why reproductive decisions are so much more complex than advocates of rational choice models for reproductive behavior would have it, as Lippman-Hand and Fraser (1979) so forcefully demonstrate. Understanding theoretic risk requires one type of inquiry; understanding materialization or its opposite, nonoccurrence, requires another.

Next, for a number of patients, the counselor's explanation of why they had a child with an anomalous condition is not satisfying. Counselors work hard in sessions to remove parental guilt for their children's condition. They explain to parents (mothers) how it is natural after an affected child is born to go over every minute of a pregnancy, but that nothing they did caused the problem. For recessive conditions, where each parent contributes a gene, to remove any sense of prenatal responsibility, counselors stress to the couple what a random event the condition is, its extraordinarily low probability, its inability to be diagnosed beforehand, and the fact that we all have "bad genes." Counselors work hard to universalize, randomize, destigmatize, and discount the importance of bad genes. However, such feelings are not so easily erased for parents.

The problem lies in the kind of stories that counselors construct for patients. Counselors explain birth defects at a chromosomal or metabolic level (when they can explain them). These explanations leave parents feeling dissatisfied; as one put it, "Well, now I know what happened, but I still don't know why it happened." Nor are couples reassured when they are told that "nothing you did caused this problem." As one mother explained, "The baby came from me, so I feel that it had something to do with me."

> I bumped into a couple I had observed in a counseling session in the Nightingale cafeteria. During their session, they were assured that nothing they did had caused their child's problems. I asked them how they were doing. The mother said that she really did want to know why the defect occurred. She had trouble accepting that it was an accident—she repeated that she needed to know why, what she had done. She said that the burden of the problem was made worse by the fact that four of her girlfriends were pregnant at the same time, and they had all had normal children, so she just *had* to have a reason, she was looking for a reason. She said that it was hard to accept that it really wasn't anything that she or her husband did, that it was just one of those things— because if it was just one of those things, then why did it have to happen to them?

Couples who find the existential meaninglessness of a random statistical process an incomplete explanation fill in the unexplained "Why?" in a number of ways. Religious explanations are not uncommon:

> I am with a couple who has just had counseling for a child who recently died from anencephaly. During the session, Bill Smith explained the fetal development of the brain and spinal cord. He explained as well the role of alpha-fetal protein in development. He told the parents that this was an indication of the problem.
> Bill has left the room. I am interviewing the parents. I ask them what caused the anencephaly. The mother

answers, "God, and God takes care of his mistakes. This was a mistake, and I feel now in my mind, because I am somewhat religious, that there is an angel—the baby is with God now."

This woman's sentiments are quite common. Following discussion of the biological mechanisms to which counselors attribute cause, couples often still assign cause to divine intervention. The genetic counselors as scientific professionals doing a job in a modern hospital were allowed to beg, ignore, or consider unimportant "final" causes. Service users trying to live a life (Coles 1979) were not so fortunate. Most of the service users' assignments of cause are not so "blissful" as the one above. In interviews, parents (most usually mothers) commonly see birth defects as a sign of divine retribution. For example, when questioned about the causes of their child's problem, one mother mentioned that God was punishing her for an elective abortion she had at age sixteen, while another saw a birth defect as punishment for premarital sex.

All these feelings of guilt and punishment, their links to sex, and their expression in a hospital context are of course not accidental, in two senses. They are anchored in the concrete incidents of personal experience and supported by political theory. Feminist writing about women's encounters with the profession of medicine have an underlying, unifying theme: the appropriation of ownership of women's experience of their own bodies by the medical profession. At Nightingale, there is little in the context—the examining room of a hospital—or the talk that is likely to reverse professional appropriation of women's ownership of their bodies. Nonetheless, with their value-neutral, nondirective stance, the genetic counselors are minimally "appropriators." They believe deeply in the privacy of reproductive decision making. They are able to provide it to those whose medical insurance status created an entitlement to privacy.

Frequently, parents talked about their "special children" as tests that God had set for them. It was clear that families of affected children did not view the event in the same set of terms that counselors used: for parents, birth defects did not happen through impersonal, probabilistic forces; they were not seen as arbitrary, accidental, anonymous statistical quirks. Particular tragedies that happened to particular families required particular explanations. The genetic counselors, of course, knew this; it was simply not relevant to their purposes when talking to service users.

When couples did not link defects to divine causes, they found explanations in more mundane ones. Most generally, mothers mentioned vague feelings, premonitions, they had about a pregnancy.

> Partly, I had a problem because this was a surprise child
> for me, and so there were times during the pregnancy
> that I just didn't know whether I was ready to have
> another one—and so, of course, you have guilt feelings. I
> think my feeling was, "This is my fault," especially since I
> didn't want him at all during the pregnancy.

Other mothers mentioned anger at their spouses or stress and tension in their lives as causes of their offspring's problems. In general, whether a birth defect was attributed to divine judgment or more secular provocations, mothers echoed nineteenth-century maternal impression theory to answer the existential questions "Why me?" and "Why my baby?" (Rosenberg 1976). Some mothers even feel guilty that the counseling they received did not resolve their guilt.

> Yes, you still blame yourself—they tell you not to, but you
> do it automatically. You build up a big bubble of
> negatives. You look at everything with hindsight. You
> wonder whether it was the painting, or the overexertion,
> or the vitamins. It seems like if everybody else has a
> normal child and you don't, there has to be a reason.

A second secular reason that mothers used to explain birth defects was obstetrical care. A large number of mothers felt their obstetrician was the source of their child's problems.

> You tend to go back and think, did I do anything grossly
> different from anybody else? And going back I realize I
> really haven't—in fact, I probably did things a little better
> than a lot of people. I ate organic foods, took care of

myself, that sort of thing. I go back to the birth process—I was induced, and it didn't go rapidly. I didn't have to be induced; it was for the doctor's convenience. So I keep going back to that and think maybe if I hadn't been so impatient to have the baby . . . because he did turn dusky after birth. I still go back to that.

The mother followed a regime of ritual purity designed to produce a perfect baby (Balin 1988). This having failed, the impropriety of labor induction is used to account for the baby's health problems. Moreover, if things happened as she says they happened—and given other descriptions of obstetrics (Scully 1980)—we have little cause for doubt that the mother's attribution of fault is not unreasonable. Even those mothers who do not hold their obstetricians responsible for their child's problems express considerable anger over the way they were managed after it was obvious that a defective child had been born. How women were treated immediately after the birth of a child with an obvious defect remained a source of anger and hurt.

For a number of parents, the probabilistic-mechanistic view of birth defects put forward by genetic counselors failed to convince because they were certain that their problems were caused by environmental teratogens. Even after counseling reassured them that nothing they did contributed to a child's problems, these couples found it hard to be convinced that the birth defect their child experienced and the chemicals they were exposed to were unrelated. Weekend gardeners, oil-refinery workers, ingesters of over-the-counter medications before pregnancy—all assigned the cause of their problems to these exposures to largely unknown risk.

The couples were able to dispense with the counselors' reassurances because, as they put it, things that were harmful in pregnancy were "being discovered all the time." Many couples express feelings similar to those expressed in the interview below, in which a couple explain why they are neither surprised nor convinced by the counselors' ruling out the husband's exposure to Agent Orange as a cause for fetal loss in pregnancy or two children born with birth defects:

Husband: It's very difficult to really realize the impact of everything. You get different groups that have been subject to treatment by certain chemicals, and years later they are finding problems with their children. I think we are going to go on and on finding a lot more problems. And no one is ever going to take responsibility. I don't think—I very seriously doubt—whether there will ever be any conclusive studies that show this is influenced by that— that this is caused by that.

Wife: As long as there is a monetary value put on it, as long as there are lawsuits and people trying to get money out of it.

Husband: No, it's not only that. I think, you know, probably in the last ten years, the rash of malpractice suits that doctors have had—I think that is going to limit them. Someone is not going to be a maverick and go out on a limb and say, "I have done this study and this is my conclusion." I think their conclusions are going to be very conservative conclusions.

Wife: That is what we were afraid of here. That even if they did find a connection, we weren't going to hear it from them, from a large institution. Even if the doctors wanted really, like he said, to be a maverick and really stick their necks out—their jobs, their research is involved. . . . My nightmare was that they had the results of the tests, and they linked it directly to Agent Orange, yet they had to put it all before a board because it is an institution. And then they found out that the government or Dow Chemical or something—they're the biggest contributors to the hospital—I mean they were my nightmares.

In a somewhat paradoxical way, genetic counselors reinforce these beliefs when they point out how much remains to be discovered, how many questions at present lack definitive answers, how "there are some problems that we may never have an explanation for." The methods used by couples to account for birth defects are not unlike the "lay epidemiology" that Brown and Mickelson (1990) discover in use among those in toxic environments. In the genetics counseling clinic, however, there is no geographic concentration. As a result, there is little likelihood that, like the site-specific victims of environmental disaster, those who are victims of subtle biochemical ones will be able to attract the scientific allies who might give their lay epidemiological reasoning respectability. In addition to corporate interests, genetic counselors are also assumed to be covering up for obstetrical or pediatric negligence.

In the end, perhaps the most ironic result of genetic counseling is that a process designed to support couples in their reproductive decision making, to insure their autonomy, leaves them isolated and overwhelmed with the burden of decision making. A couple talks about the "burden" of decision-making:

> The husband of a couple whose child has died from a genetic defect is reflecting on the counseling.
>
> *Husband:* They kind of, no, we handled the situation pretty much ourselves. We were always given the information, the options were pretty much sketched for us, but left open.
> *Wife:* Sometimes we wish we weren't the ones who had to make the decisions.
> *Husband:* Yeah, but that's pretty much the bottom line. We are the ones who make the final decision.
> *Wife:* Getting the information, that's the best we can do. What more can you do? But the decision is a burden.

The burden of decision making is, of course, not the only one that the genetic counselors leave to patients. For some, there are additionally the burdens of servicing a child with special needs: finding the right programs, arranging payment for them, and still maintaining some equipoise. All of these burdens counselors acknowledge, but they also pass them to others: social workers and support groups. Moreover, the genetic counselors at Nightingale do not follow up to see how well others have managed with these problems. This is not necessarily a criticism: the absence of regular follow-up lessens the amount of official surveillance. Privacy is preserved.

There is one final burden that parents also have to face: their own impotence and powerlessness to change the situation. This requires accepting the limits on their children's development, despite finding the best infant-stimulation programs, procuring the best support services, and providing the best parenting. It requires accepting the limits of the possible. As one mother put it, "All my life I try to help my daughter. I, I hope to find some way to help her. And now I can't. It's not possible."

In the end, this impotence overwhelms some parents; their children become a source of "chronic sorrow" (Olshansky 1973), their original loss is reexperienced as each developmental milestone fails to be reached.[14] For the genetic counselors' part, their own impotence to fix what could not be fixed often overwhelmed them. Finally, watching all this as a witness, being asked to help and not knowing how, overwhelmed me as well. I was often angry at the genetic counselors both for what they failed to do for patients and what they expected me to do for both them and their patients. Finally, I felt some sort of cosmic anger that there was so much random and contingent pain and suffering. I was overwhelmed and then paralyzed by the limits of rational understanding.

14. This is, of course, not the only response. The success of support groups for parents of "special children" reveals another mode of response. Of course "chronic sorrow" and "successful normalization" are only analytically distinct. Empirically, it is possible to imagine the same person having each feeling quite closely connected in time.

3

COUNSELING AS A
MOP-UP SERVICE

The last chapter focused on the work of genetic counselors in its most mundane form: seeing patients in weekly clinic. But to focus on clinic work alone—on its successes, its imperfections, and its failures—even if this work is the "core task" of genetic counselors, commits a grave sampling error: It mistakes a part for the whole. However central clinic is to counselors' work, it occupies only a small part of their time budget as both workers and as clinicians. Clinic takes but one afternoon a week. Group and individual preparation for cases requires at a minimum, another half day and at a maximum, another day and a half for preparation, or "story-fixing."

The everyday clinical work of genetic counselors takes other forms as well. This chapter analyzes one of those forms, routine requests for consultations. It places genetic counselors in a hierarchy within the medical division of labor in the modern hospital, explores how counselors define their obligations to colleagues, and talks about the work that genetic counselors do for their colleagues. In particular, it defines counseling as a devalued professional status.

Counseling in the Medical Division of Labor

As Hughes (1971) first pointed out, the routinized practice of referral and consultation among colleagues in a hospital is a way of sharing troubles, spreading risk, and distributing guilt for untoward outcomes. Although formally equal, physicians in the hospital division of labor are arrayed in a hierarchy by two major determinants. The first is technical prowess. Those with highly specialized skills, the application of which promises dramatic "saves"—specialists like neonatologists, oncologists, pediatric surgeons—stand at the top of the hierarchy.[1] The second, less powerful determinant is everyday clinical decision-making capabilities. The genetic counselors, having nothing special to offer save talk and elective abortion, and having no primary care responsibilities for patients, are at the bottom of the medical status hierarchy. In Abbott's (1981) terms, the work of genetic counselors is professionally impure, full of social mess, and hence of low intraprofessional status.

A number of concrete indicators mark the low status of genetic counseling in the hierarchy of professional prestige at Nightingale Children's Center. First, for both medical students and pediatric residents at Nightingale, clinical genetics was a clinical elective— exposure to it was not required.[2] Undergraduate and postgraduate students rarely elected to spend time learning to do what genetic counselors did. During the three years of this research, only three students did rotations on genetics, and each of them claimed it was a slow service. It was not, however the slowness that bothered the students, who often chose electives for that reason alone, to get a breather after more punishing rotations. What bothered students more was the failure to take away something useful. In addition, although the service did offer regular fellowships for advanced training in clinical genetics, the two physicians who availed themselves of this opportunity spent most of their time in the laboratory learn-

1. Among clinicians in established subspecialties, there are *geneticists*— individuals trying to make the next therapeutic step by new genetic techniques. These people should not be confused with genetic counselors; they are on different career paths. They have no need of the occupational title *genetic counselor*. Genetic technologies may advance in the hospital hierarchy without genetic counselors gaining anything but more work at the same devalued status.

2. The low place of clinical genetics in the later years of medical education contrasts sharply with its esteemed place in the first two, or "basic education," years of medical training at Nightingale Medical School. Genetics is a required basic science course in the first two years of training at Nightingale, or (to hedge a bit) this was so at the time of this research. One message about human genetics that students could extract from the curricular structure involving human genetics was that it was basic science that was clinically irrelevant.

ing research techniques. Despite trying, one of these physicians was unable to secure employment as a genetic counselor; the other had little interest in doing so, the genetics fellowship was a bit of credential-building for another career path.

The low esteem of the physician/genetic counselor at Nightingale Children's Center was mirrored nationally in a number of ways. There is now, and was at the time of this research, both scant opportunity for physician training as a genetic counselor and, as the experience of Nightingale Children's Fellows demonstrated, few institutional positions available for those with the requisite training. In most institutions which provide genetic counseling, the physician/genetic counselor either never existed or has been replaced by the graduate of a two-year program awarding the Master of arts in genetic counseling. This has not happened at Nightingale Children's Center. Looking at the work the genetic counselors of Nightingale do for their colleagues may tell us why.

Before turning to that, it is worth noting that the counselors were themselves aware that they were in an anomalous position. On the one hand, they were aware of the glamour that was attached to genetics because of recent breakthroughs, many of which promised new clinical applications; and they were even proud to claim some of these new discoveries as their own.[3] On the other hand, they were aware that they were viewed by their colleagues as a clinical backwater. In the hospital, genetic counselors were not (in the housestaff slang of the time) "major players." Although this collegial evaluation stung their pride, because of the absence of definitive therapeutic interventions, they were unable to do very much to combat it.

When counselors spoke of their roles, they tended to look back wistfully to a preceding generation of geneticists who were able to unite excellence both at the bench and the bedside. These role models whose missionary zeal helped establish the field repre-

3. The genetic counselors were aware that there was a frontier in applied clinical genetics and that they were not on it. The frontier is, however, not a counseling frontier—it is a surgical frontier and a scientific one. Genetic therapies will attract more than a few recruits to a variety of subspecialties. Fetal surgery will appeal to many. But counseling as a distinct and primary job task will appeal to few physicians.

sented a no-longer attainable ideal to the individuals at Night-ingale.[4] With the explosion of knowledge in genetics, the current counselors did not see how it was possible that the accomplishments of the giants of the first generation could be matched in the present:

> I am talking with Bill Smith about the balance between research and clinical work. He says, "I don't think there is a person that can do excellent Ph.D.-quality research and decent clinical genetics practice and combine the two. Maybe once, but not any more. I think a person falls short on one of the two things. Me, being a nonexcellent bench person, I don't fit the model. The bench people, being nonexcellent clinicians, don't fit the model. I have become very, very frustrated with the whole concept. Now I figure, as long as I do my work, as long as I do it well, as long as I'm careful, I'm making a contribution."

When Palmer replaced Berger as chief of the service, there was some hope that Palmer would use his power at Nightingale (he was also, at the time, chairman of pediatrics) to improve the status of the service.[5]

> Bill Smith is talking about possible benefits from Berger's departure and Palmer's arrival. This is hard for him to do since he was close to Berger and is having some difficulty accepting his moving on. He says, "Maybe this man can do something for the division (clinical genetics). Give it something that it didn't have before because it was never given the respect that maybe it should or shouldn't have. If it gets his full attention—and he p.r.'s, which is

---

4. Here is one place where particularities make a difference. At another institution, there most likely would have been another set of ideals and aspirations.

5. In terms of *humble and proud* and *group identifications,* the genetic counseling unit shifted multiple ways with the replacement of Berger by Palmer. Berger was a proud link to clinical genetics and the past at Nightingale. He gave the group a "cosmopolitan pride." This identity was damaged by his departure. Palmer replaced cosmopolitan pride with local pride. They were now more intimately linked to the top of the organizational chart. But as I've mentioned, the genetic counselors were cosmopolitans; local pride did not conform with their ideals.

something that he knows how to do—than maybe it will build the unit up in the institution."

But this attention is something that even the division of clinical genetics' most active physician member is ambivalent about. When speaking about the division's lack of respect in the hospital, Bill Smith is unsure whether this respect is something that it should or shouldn't have. If respect comes, it will not be for what the workers in the division accomplish. Rather, collegial respect will come from Palmer's p.r. efforts, and then only if it gets his full attention. Not only that, the respect itself will not be generated by "good, efficient, useful service," which all physicians would respect, but rather by a kind of "selling," which is inherently distasteful to their scientific norms.

Further, although their lack of status rankles them, being in a clinical backwater offers advantages to both Bill Smith and Albert Samuels. For Bill Smith, the absence of primary care responsibilities allows him some control over his life-style. It allows him to combine family and a professional career with a minimum of stress.[6] At the same time, the cognitive complexity of genetics problems pleases him, as does the absence of decision-making responsibility.

> I am talking with Bill Smith about his decision to go into
> genetic counseling. He answered, "I couldn't stand
> internal medicine, with all the people falling apart, and
> you just patch. I said, 'What do I like?' and I like this. I like
> getting a fascinoma[7] like you have never seen, then
> spending all the time in the library, figuring them out,
> and so on. . . . Feeling not overwhelmed and having
> enough time either to know or to know that nobody
> knows what it is."

6. I do not want to appear unsympathetic here. The juggling required of Bill Smith to meet conflicting obligations was great in itself, as it is for many in all lines of work. I am placing the stress of personal and professional demands of physicians on a continuum. For physicians, even the minimally stressful end of this continuum may contain a large amount of stress. Little attention has been paid to the private lives of professionals; for two useful exceptions to this rule, see Broadhead (1983) and Gerber (1983).

7. Doctor argot for "fascinating case."

For Smith, the emphasis is not so much on what is done for patients as what is found out about them. Now Bill takes comfort in the fact that he is able to help residents who are overwhemed (as he once was) by infants with multiple anomalies. What Bill likes best is a problem with a clear answer and enough time to find it. Most of the time, his work as a genetic counselor provides this.

Samuels chose to be a genetic counselor because it allowed him to sustain his identity as a physician while pursuing a research career:

> Well, I was interested in science, but I went to medical school. It (genetics) was an area of medicine that had the least pressing medical care situation, plus it was the research area that I wanted to be in; it would give me the opportunity to do research, so it seemed logical. I am primarily interested in research, but I was trained as a physician. I would never accept a position that did not involve some patient care, although I don't choose to be involved in day-to-day decision making. I knew I would find the general practice of medicine intellectually stultifying, and I didn't see that any other subspecialty area of medicine would allow me to do the kind of research that I want to do, would allow me the time.

To put it as his colleague sometimes did, "Samuels fusses around in his lab, and nobody—okay maybe a few people—understand what he is doing." For either Smith or Samuels, more duties that involved clinical decision making and the attendant responsibility would disturb the balance that their limited clinical roles allowed them as they pursued other, more primary, interests.

Of the physicians on the genetics counseling team, only Joseph Giordano, a high-risk obstetrician doing "exciting," "world-class," "important" work in the field of prenatal medicine, had significant primary care responsibilities. Only for Giordano was genetic counseling a secondary rather than a primary clinical task. It was a matter of courtesy that he met with "amnio" patients during clinic, but administratively speaking, "amnio" patients were, at the time of this study, a group separate from "genetic counseling" ones. Giordano never identified himself as a genetic counselor; for him, prenatal diagnostic procedures were an adjunct to a large clinical practice. Genetics was a supplement to what he did, not the thing itself.

In requesting consultations and making referrals, treating physicians are asking for help. They are seeking ideas for diagnosis and treatment when they have run out of ideas themselves, or they are seeking to transfer responsibility for their clinical problems to another service, a practice known to residents as *turfing*.[8] Against these shopfloor beliefs and practices for seeking help from colleagues, enlisting genetic counselors appears peculiar. After all, genetic counselors rarely provide information that has any direct relevance for treatment; and with no primary care responsibilities, there is no hope that the genetic counselor will somehow take the referring physician's problems off his hands. So why do other physicians at Nightingale Children's Center seek help from genetic counselors? And what kind of help do they seek?

Mopping-Up

We already know that the work of genetic counseling involves a significant amount of social dirty work. Given their position in the intraprofessional prestige hierarchy at Nightingale, it should come as no surprise that this is true, as well, for the work they perform at the behest of their colleagues. The genetic counselors are in the basement of the prestige hierarchy, and it is to the basement that other physicians go to find help to "mop up" messy situations.

There are three common messy situations in which genetic counselors find themselves routinely involved because of the "normal, natural troubles" of colleagues providing hospital care.[9] On

8. For a fictional account of the practice of turfing, see Shem (1978). For a discussion of the competition among physicians for patients, the attempt to expand rather than contract professional turf, see De Santis (1980). For basic ideas about turf, competition, and professionals, see Goode (1960).

9. There is a long history of studying normal, natural troubles within sociology. This study merges a Hughesian concern for "rough edges, routines, and emergencies," and specific shopfloor remedies with a more ethnomethodologically located concern for the inherent, essential reflexivity of any social construction of reality. Within the sociology of medicine, consider Sudnow's (1967) account of "passing on" as a normal, natural source of trouble in hospitals. In looking at police work, Bittner (1967a, 1967b) focuses on the normal, natural troubles of the skid-row policeman.

these occasions the organizational place of genetic counseling puts them in line for referrals. This place is not exalted, and these referrals do not represent a show of deference to superior expertise. In fact, in the language of residents, such referrals are successful *dumps* in the game of *turfing* onerous and unwanted problems and responsibilities. The first type of referral involves counselors in their core task, counseling patients, but under very trying conditions immediately following the death of a child.

Pediatrics and obstetrics are two areas of modern hospital care not routinely associated with death. So much is this the case that it is often said to attract recruits to these fields. As genetic counselors well know (and their sociological shadow soon learns), low-probability events happen, and with a large enough population base, they happen with some regularity. Two to three percent of all infants are born with significant birth anomalies. Because of the regionalization of specialized pediatric care and triage, many of these receive extensive treatment in the various specialized units of Nightingale Children's Center, most prominently, the Neonatal Intensive Care Unit. Even with the best available care, some of these children die. When this happens, sometimes those in charge of care are not able to give parents more of an explanation than "His lungs were just too immature" or "There were problems with the heart." They are unable to give full explanations because they lack complete data; for example, data from pathology which would pinpoint a reason for a child's problem or demise. At the same time, even with incomplete data, neonatologists overload parents with pathophysiological detail. Infant death is an event that needs more processing than a neonatal intensive care unit provides.

Even if this were not the case, a comprehensive explanation of infant death to a neonatologist is not a full story to a parent who is vitally interested in the critical item that the neonatologist's tale leaves out: the risk of recurrence, the probability of lightning striking twice. Invariably, the parents of these children are referred to the genetic counselors. Ideally, the counselors are introduced to the parents while the child is still alive and then counsel them at clinic following a child's death at the parent's initiative, a signal of a readiness to hear and listen. Often this ideal is not met, and the counselors' session with parents is also their initial meeting. Much as the counselors pressed the genetic associate and me to mop up patients who flooded emotionally, neonatologists and oncologists use genetic counselors to mop up the feelings of bereaved parents.

I am ready to join Bill Smith in a counseling session with the Delberts. I am doing so at Bill's request. He also asked me not to gather a consent, and I agreed. Bill had characterized the Delberts' counseling story as having a bad case of the "vagues." Bill has questions about the Delberts' cognitive capacity. He describes them as borderline functional. He states that if they found a stamped letter by a mailbox, they would give it to the authorities rather than mail it. When we enter the treatment room, we are a chair short because the Delberts have mounted a portable tape-recorder on a chair. As Bill introduces me as "his associate," it occurs to me that he may have underestimated the Delbert's capabilities.

Bill begins the session by apologizing for the delay today (we are forty-five minutes late due to two "stat" consults), for the delay in setting up this meeting (it is six months since the child's death; the session has had to be rescheduled twice because lab work was not complete), and for the fact that even now not all the results are in from neuropathology.

Bill begins by eliciting from the Delberts their chief concern, which is fear of recurrence. He responds to this curiously: "You should realize that it is not just me talking, that I have talked to lots of other doctors in the hospital, and this is what we have come up with. . . . I am going over this because at the time Paul was here, I remember that we didn't get to talk too much. Everything centered around his immediate medical problems, which were considerable. I don't really remember us having a chance to talk then."

The Delberts agree, and Bill, rather than turning to the concern for recurrence that he has just elicited from the Delberts, begins to take a history of Paul's problems from his parents. This he does, despite the fact that he has just reviewed Paul's humongous chart in preparation for the Delbert's visit.

In the middle of the session, Bill is called from the room, and I am left alone with the Delberts.[10] Exquisitely uncomfortable, I make small talk about housing in Tulsa, where this couple will soon relocate.

Bill returns to the room and begins to give the Delberts the story on their recurrence risk. He stated that from his point of view, choking was the most prominent thing about Paul medically. He went on, ". . . one explanation stands out: G-syndrome. Children with G-syndrome tend to have unexplained choking episodes, and their ears sort of turn outward, and their eyes tend to be far apart. These were all features of Paul's."

Bill explains he was on the phone that morning "to Montana" with the "world's leading expert on G-syndrome and the person who discovered it." He reported that there was no way to eliminate the possibility of G-syndrome without examining the parents and looking at Paul's medical records.

He then asked the parents if they had pictures of Paul, "especially any close to the face," so that he could send them with the records to Montana.

Bill then explained the recurrence risk: "Now for the chances of this happening again. We don't really know. We do know from experience that a certain number of congenital problems go unexplained and that 6 percent of those mothers have second children with birth defects. So if we don't ever figure this out, the odds are 6 per cent. Of if it's G-syndrome, the odds are 50 percent for having

10. Bill's exit here is yet another marker of how unlike counseling and how much more like a standard clinical encounter counseling sessions are. It is hard to imagine such interruptions in routine versions of counseling: psychotherapy, psycho-analysis, marital or family therapy, or groupwork. Yet such interruptions are fre-quent in genetic counseling. In this case, Bill was, as I later found out, yanked from the room to examine an infant whose physical findings on exam posed some ques-tions for Samuels.

another child like Paul, because G-syndrome has a 50
percent recurrence risk."

He then asked for the parents' assistance in "trying to
get a definitive answer." He then took some
measurements of the parent's head circumference and
inner and outer pupillary distance to forward to Montana.

The "vagues" of the Delberts created a number of concrete problems for Bill Smith—How could she give them a recurrence risk
without a diagnostic label? Further, the label is not inconsequential.
With one label, the "reproductive risk," as the counselors call it,
doubled; with the other, it was magnified more than sixteen times.
He faced as well the problem of helping the Delberts manage their
grief. About this he also had the vagues.

He had, however, worked out a number of steps for eliciting and
containing grief within a single session. Bill's strategy was shared by
the other members of the workgroup and is what they understood
mopping up to mean operationally. Mopping-up visits were often
for clients a last official visit in a major episode of pediatric ill-
ness. Hence, the genetic counselors often had to account for any
"glitches" in service during what were very eventful and complex
hospitalizations. To the Delberts, waiting for the past six months (as
well as for Bill today) was one such glitch. Encouraging the Delberts
to talk is not unrisky for the counselors. Considering the stress of
infant death, genetic counselors are likely to be caught in "affect
storms," given the turbulence of parental feeling.

Moreover, some of this risk was routinely created by the counselor's colleagues. For example, delays like the Delberts' in getting
the results from pathology for postmortem follow-ups were recurrent and apparently intractable, a routine feature of mop-up visits.
The genetic counselors viewed the problem as, in part, a reflection
of their low status and the lack of urgency associated with postmortem results. Although vexed by the slowness themselves, the genetic counselors invariably protected the pathologists in front of
parents, stressing the complexity of the lab work. Parents complained bitterly about these delays in scheduling. They said that
they felt "like I lost four months of my life" or that they had "been
on pins and needles for a long time now." The genetic counselors

acknowledge when they are with parents that this is unfortunate, but among themselves they express some relief that the parents are less likely to be "raw" after a long delay.

As the last specialists seen at Nightingale, the genetic counselors close up cases. They provide once again an explanation for what happened. But they do more than simply mop up. As those that see all the children born with significant birth anomalies, all of God's mistakes, they witness for their colleagues, much as I witnessed for them. Through this witnessing, they accomplish a number of things. First, their presence helps relieve their colleagues of guilt, blame, and responsibility. Second, they serve the hospital as a whole as organizational "shock absorbers." They allow their colleagues a place to send their troubles; having that, these colleagues need not miss any more beats than they have to when action goes awry. This is not to say that those that care for these infants who die do not deal at all with parental needs; the assertion is more limited than that. Genetic counseling as a service provides an arena for turfing these needs, for separating the parents from their hospital experience.

The counseling of bereaved parents is not the only way that counselors mop up for their colleagues; a second type of routine consultation requires cleaning up a different sort of mess. Nightingale has many children whose complex problems involve the coordinated efforts of physicians in multiple specialties. These colleagues do not always get along with each other, nor do they always give parents consistent stories. These mixed signals create problems for housestaff at Nightingale, who find themselves confused about treatment priorities or about how best to manage parents. In these situations housestaff often call upon counselors.[11] By requesting consults in these cases, housestaff try to enlist counselors as mediators in conflicts between specialties or as communicators to make sure that parents are dealt with effectively.

11. The genetic counselors are not the only professionals who could be called upon this way. Consultation is a general device to resolve conflict. The universe of others that housestaff can call on is limited only by their resourcefulness and the sensitivities of the attending, supervisory authorities. This consult strategy is used by residents in all specialties. What changes is who is being asked to mediate disagreements through consultation.

When I show up at Bill Smith's office, he tells me that I missed a really "zoo-ey" day yesterday (a teaching day for me). What had made it zooey was that he had a lot of unscheduled patient contact, in addition to lecturing the required medical school course and planning for the impending grant site visit, which "Berger was getting very antsy about."

He described one of these unscheduled consults in great detail. He said that he had had a request from an intern to see the parents of a child with Goldenhar's syndrome. Everything was wrong with the child, he added; it had every feature of the syndrome.

He said that although usually he liked talking with parents—it was the part of his job he liked best—on this occasion he felt very uncomfortable. I replied, "No wonder, you always have such good news for them."

He protested, "Well, for these parents I did have good news. I told them that the child, for all its problems, was not retarded, and that there was no recurrence risk, so they were happy."

I asked if he had such good news, why was he distressed. It turns out the source of his discomfort resides in how the consult came about. He said that an intern had sought him out and said that he had some parents that Bill "just had to talk to today." He had protested that there was no emergency and he was swamped. The intern kept insisting that he just had to see the parents right away. He asked why? The intern explained, "Because one attending won't deal with the parents, won't give them a full story, and the other attending is boorish."

So Bill Smith said that he told the intern, "Well, look, if you get them all in one room, and you let the boorish one speak, I'll cushion whatever he says."

He then complained to me, "So that's how people look at us—they think we're a mop-up service, a cushion, for everything else that goes on around here."

While the physicians at Nightingale Children's Center may try to employ counselors this way, the counselors occasionally try to construct some boundaries around these practices. They sometimes do not give patients full stories but send them back to referring physicians with questions they think should be appropriately addressed by treating physicians.

> Albert Samuels mentions that he has just been made very uncomfortable by a chance encounter with Mrs. Castleberry in the hospital cafeteria. The Castleberrys have a child with prune-belly syndrome. He had counseled the Castleberrys two weeks ago. During the session, they had asked him what their child's prognosis was, because the surgeons had never discussed this with the parents. Samuels had told them that this was something they had best talk about with the surgeons treating their child.
>
> When he saw the mother, he asked about the child. The mother said the child was going home today but that she realized how little time the child had to live. Samuels was made very uncomfortable by the mother's affect. He described her as half-laughing, half-crying. Samuels said he felt like a "heel" bumping into the mother. He said it was one of those situations where "I knew something that you didn't know, and now you know it too."

Samuels did not avoid telling the Castleberrys the full story because he was unaware of it, but because of his sense that such momentous bad news should be conveyed by treating physicians. By funneling the Castleberrys back to the surgeons with encouragement to ask their question, he was at one and the same time reassuring them that it was a legitimate question, while trying to force his colleagues to live up to their role obligations. Quite regularly, after consults with the parents of sick infants, the counselors express some amazement at the difficulty parents have in extracting a full story from treating physicians. They also express some anger at the way their colleagues assume that they will do their dirty work for them. However sympathetic they are to patients' problems, the genetic counselors limit their intervention. They do not orchestrate disclosure as they do when residents ask for help.

Consultations with residents are not only for mop-up. Residents also use genetic counselors to provide "spot lessons" in the diagnosis of birth defects. Here the consult parallels the exchange relationship that Miller (1970) first described among housestaff and attendings at Boston City Hospital. Housestaff, when presented with diagnostic problems in children, consult the counselors. The counselors receive a chance to look at interesting clinical material. The housestaff receive quick, didactic lessons in what to look for in this or that syndrome. Specialty consults, generally, are used by housestaff in this way to supplement their formal training, to combat the sense (universal among housestaff) that their own educational needs are secondary to the hospital's need for a cheap source of labor for the most routine of physicianly ministrations, and to increase their confidence level in their assessment of patient problems.

Whatever information residents glean from these consultations often appears secondary to their value as support. The counselor's presence establishes that, yes, this is a "funny" baby; no, we don't know why; no, we can't say anything for certain about the baby's future development; and yes, it is difficult to know what to say to parents under these situations. Residents gain from these exchanges something often missing in their interactions with supervising attending faculty—the ear of a sympathetic colleague. Here again the genetic counselors act as witnesses to how difficult it is to be a resident at Nightingale, where the expectations for professional conduct by supervisors are both unforgiving and all-encompassing.

It is not just the attending physicians and housestaff at Nightingale Children's that use the genetic counselors. Community pediatricians also use the counselors to deliver bad news. By doing so, they can preserve their relationships with families and let the genetic counselors, whose involvement with parents is at best episodic, act as the "heavies."

Al Samuels is discussing many of the routine referrals that come to the clinic, cases where community pediatricians

could make a diagnosis but choose not to. "Most private
physicians don't deal adequately—don't feel adequate—
to dispense this information most of the time. Most of the
time they don't want to, because this is bad news; that is
why we get a lot of the Down's syndrome cases. The
physician who is going to care for the child for the rest of
its childhood doesn't want to be the heavy; so we can be
the heavy, and he can just care for the colds, because that
is what he is going to do anyway. And why should he drop
these terrible bombs? Most of the time they don't know
the information, anyway. So that's what we do."

As consultants, then, the genetic counselors mop up those who
have been bombed by misfortune and then drop some bombs
themselves as a courtesy to colleagues who do not want to be associated with the psychological terrorism inherent in revealing some
unyielding biomedical truth.

Gatekeepers without Turf

Attending neonatologists also use counseling services as the residents do. They, too, show counselors their problems. But their requests are more weighty than those made by residents. Attending
neonatologists call upon counselors to sanction treatment or not.
Needless to say, the withdrawal of treatment from severely ill neonates is a complex issue. At Nightingale Children's Center, these
problems are made even more difficult by a significant number of
physicians who espouse a right-to-life ideology.

The neonatologists at Nightingale understand well that not initiating treatment is easier than discontinuing it once it has begun.
Even so, not initiating treatment is itself a very difficult decision.
This decision is made easier for them if a lethal genetic abnormality
which would make treatment futile is discovered. If such is the case,
neonatologists feel a decision not to treat is morally justified. Without such a finding, this decision is more difficult.

Bill Smith and Albert Samuels have been called to the
Neonatal Intensive Care Unit. The neonatologists want to
do a bone-marrow tap, rather than the more standard

venipuncture, to find out as soon as possible if a child has trisomy 18, a chromosomal abnormality which causes severe retardation and death, usually in the first year of life.

When Smith and Samuels get to the bedside, a team of hematologists has already gathered at the baby's bedside, ready to harvest the bone-marrow. Bill chases them from the bedside, explaining that he was going to look at the child, and on the basis of what he saw, they were going to do a bone-marrow or not. The hematologists left looking miffed, telling Bill to beep them if their services were needed.

Both Bill and Samuels examine the baby. They agree that although it most likely has a chromosomal problem, possibly a translocation, there is no reason to suspect trisomy 18, and therefore no reason to do a bone-marrow.

Bill calls the baby's attending and reports the findings from the exam. The attending asks Bill to "wait right there." He appears moments later.

He listens to Bill's recitation of findings on physical exams and summary diagnostic conclusions. He then asks if it is possible to rule out trisomy 18 totally without a karyotype. Bill says no. The attending says he is uncomfortable with the child on a ventilator as long as trisomy 18 is a possibility. He wants the marrow for karyotyping; does Bill agree that it is necessary for the "quickest" diagnosis? He does. The attending calls hematology.

Samuels, Smith, and I retreat to a side room. Samuels began to complain to Bill Smith: "This is ridiculous. Everybody can see this is a bad baby. They're just keeping it alive to make a diagnosis . . ." Samuels keeps complaining about misallocated resources, unnecessary procedures, and about treating attending anxiety rather than the patient.

At this last comment, Bill Smith grows testy and barks back at Samuels, "Enough, already, I know you think it's a bad baby. I think it's a bad baby, too. But that's not the point. It's not the question. Look you want to put on a green scrub suit and take care of these patients, fine. Then you can decide what tests need to be done or not. I am a consultant. He told me that he would be helped by the test, and I ordered it for him. I said okay."

Samuels said that it was a matter of judgment, and that he disagreed with the attending's in this case.

Bill Smith agreed, saying, "Yes, it is a matter of judgment—and if you want to make the final judgment, then you have to take care of the patients. Otherwise, it's my job as a consultant to help attendings in whatever way they ask for."

Samuels, it is worth noting, disagrees with the handling of this case and not with the definition of consultant responsibility.

Genetic counselors are as nonintrusive with the decision making of their colleagues as they are with their patients. In this case, their actions serve as a warrant for attendings to claim clinical autonomy in ordering tests and treatment. Here their nonjudgmental stance contributes to procedures and treatment that they believe unwarranted for other prognostic reasons. (The baby's skull was positive on a transillumination test [light from a flashlight beamed on one side of the skull and visible on the other], indicating an incompletely formed brain.) Nonetheless, however uncomfortable they are with the decision to perform the bone-marrow and, ultimately, to treat this infant, neither counselor raises these concerns with the attending in neonatology.

Once neonatologists have diagnostic information from genetic counselors, they use it in formulating treatment plans. Very often, they request the counselor's presence at conferences with parents to present the genetic information. In these sessions, the counselors' role as information givers is paramount. Further, the gap between what they report, what is then planned, and how they feel about it is sometimes very striking:

Bill Smith is meeting with Francois Marceau, an attending in neonatology, just prior to meeting with the Doughertys, who have a baby girl with an unbalanced translocation, a rare chromosomal abnormality, and a serious heart defect. There is some uncertainty and disagreement about how to manage the child. Bill explains to Marceau that the translocation is rare (he could only uncover five cases in the literature) and that a poor prognosis is attached to this defect.

Marceau listens and says that this information changes his thinking about the baby; that he wants to give it "didge and diuretics" to keep it comfortable but is reluctant to cath it or repair the underlying defect. After stating what he thinks of as the minimum care necessary in this situation, Marceau adds, "I also have to consider my staff. I can't, for instance promise that if the baby stops breathing, no one will bag it. I'm not on the floor twenty-four hours a day. I think there's a psychological reflex if a baby stops breathing, to bag it. I can't promise what my staff will do."

Marceau and Bill Smith agree that he will present the chromosomal picture, and Marceau will discuss treatment with the Doughertys.

After they make their presentations, Mr. Dougherty begins to talk: "We've talked about this, and we're both ready to raise a retarded child if it will live. We've also talked about heroics and have misgivings. If it's Nature's course for the baby to survive, we can accept that responsibility. But we don't want any heroic measures taken to extend the baby's life . . ."

Marceau responds, "Fine, good, we're all thinking along the same lines, because I'm very comfortable with no surgery and no catherization, just making her comfortable with didge and diuretics. . . . Right now let me share my thinking with you as a physician, because I'm responsible for the people around here every day. Didge and diuretics will extend her life, but to me and my staff, giving it to her is not heroic. It is the same as feeding her."

The father asks for more information on the child's prognosis. Marceau equivocates, "There are a lot of possibilities. I don't know what the probabilities for each one are."

The conference goes on, with the father objecting to the treatment plan, and Marceau assuring him that it is a minimum plan, that this treatment is really nontreatment. Reluctantly the parents agree to give their child digitalis and diuretics.

After the meeting, Bill calls me aside. He is very disturbed. He says to me, "I don't think Marceau was very straight with those parents. He wants to give the baby didge and diuretics, and he wasn't listening to what they were saying. They were saying that they would like nature to take its course. Here you have this situation, you have this tragedy: it's terrible, it's hard to recover from, it's just miserable, whatever. You have this situation where nature is ready to take its course; but, if you go ahead and intervene, who knows? You may save the baby, which is the last thing anybody really wants in this situation. Here, the father was saying 'I've got to think of my family. I don't want this tragedy to ruin my family. I don't know if we can really handle it,' and Marceau says, 'Sure, we want what you want.' And all the time he's planning to save the baby. I don't think he played very straight with that family."

Evident in the handling of this patient is Bill Smith's distress at the way that Marceau managed the Doughertys. At no time in the conference did he suggest an alternative to Marceau's plan for the treatment of the Doughertys' child, nor did he mention to Marceau privately any of his questions. The nondirective, expert neutrality of the genetic counselors marks their relationship with their colleagues every bit as much as it does their dealings with patients. This is so, even though here their lack of intervention serves to undermine patient autonomy, the very value that neutrality was adopted to protect.

The concern for how genetic information is used in making treatment decisions is widespread among members of the team. On occasion, members of the genetic service share Marceau's concern with the impact of nontreatment decisions on other hospital staff.

When I got to clinic, Nancy Thomas told me that there
was an infant in the hospital with trisomy 13 that I might
be interested in. The baby was born with no eyes, with
extra digits, and with other malformations associated
with this chromosomal syndrome. She reported that the
parents had decided not only that they did not want to
repair the child's oomphalecele, but they wanted the
child to die, and they were willing to do what they could
to hurry that event along. The parents had left orders that
the child not be fed. She reported that Berger was very
upset with this turn of events. In fact, it greatly reduced
the pleasure he felt in demonstrating the efficacy of skin
biopsy as a way of doing chromosomal analysis. Berger
thought it was not fair for the nurses to have to watch this
child die. Berger claimed that it was one thing for the
physicians and the parents to handle this, and quite
another for the nurses who had to deal with the infant
every day and would be the ones to watch it starve.

As upset as Berger was, he was not in any position to change the
outcome. He had provided the critical information; in fact, he was
quite proud of being able to do so, yet he was not part of the group
that had decided how this information was to be used.

This case illustrates a recurrent tension between the staff of neonatologists and the genetic counselors. Often the neonatologists
request a consultation with genetics but then request that the genetic counselors not explain their findings to the parents. The genetic counselors find this practice unacceptable at the same time
that they accede to the requests of the neonatologists.

Samuels is explaining to me some of the frustrations in
dealing with the neonatology unit, which have just come
to a head once again because the geneticists were asked
to examine a child with a "big" foot but not to meet with
the parents. "Now the problem, I gather, is that in the
past, when many consults have been called on patients
with defects, the neonatologists have interpreted the fact
of a lot of physicians coming to see the patient and then
talking to the parents—who have just given birth and are

therefore in a somewhat confused state—they have not looked upon that in a positive way. They [the neonatologists] have considered that more confusion than light to the parents' understanding of the child. . . . And so they have decided that they will be the sole dispensers of information. And this is looked upon by the consultants as unacceptable because they need information from the parents and because they are being belittled by being put into a secondary position. Here, the neonatologists are shirking their responsibility by making the decision that they want to shield the parents, which is inappropriate because the parents are already concerned. What they should have done is explain to the family what is being done, introduce the consultant, and then that's that. It's wrong of the neonatologists to have made the decision for the parents that we shouldn't discuss it [the big foot] with them because it was insignificant. Their attitude [the neonatologists] I think was that the child was a newborn, the mother is just getting acquainted with her baby, she should be, she is, excited by the fact of having a baby. The problem isn't life-threatening or really significant, so let the mother and child interact and forget about it. But that is easier said than done. And it's not their decision. They shirked a responsibility. It's bad medicine."

While Samuels was as unhappy with the management of this case as Berger was with the one preceding it, it is interesting that he agreed to practice what he thought of as "bad medicine." This, if nothing else, is an indicator of the relative power of neonatologists and genetic counselors within the status hierarchy at Nightingale. Subordination in a hierarchy involves the support of policies and commission of actions that the individual might prefer to be different.

The genetic counselors act as gatekeepers of outpatient services by referring their patients to specialty clinics, parent support groups, and social service agencies. Inside the hospital, the genetic counselors control access to resources as well. Genetic diagnosis often determines how much care a child will or will not get. But in all of this, the counselors are gatekeepers without turf; their gatekeeping decisions neither expand nor contract the service's own workload. Once their decisions are made, they control the flow of patients to others but do not influence the amount of work that they themselves do.

Although formally equal, the counselors never exercise any of those prerogatives one might expect when colleagues disagree. They do not push their own point of view. They do not even use the device of the gentle question to get their colleagues to reconsider courses of action which they consider ill-advised. The counselors adopt instead what they call a "consultant ethos," which, for them, means providing colleagues with whatever it is they want.

Nonetheless, they fret about the parents who look as if they are heading for troubles that the counselors themselves can do little to prevent.

> Bill Smith had just met with the parents of the child with trisomy 13 who have given orders that their child not be fed. [The orders were ignored by the neonatology service]. He is reporting on his meeting at the postclinic conference. Bill said that most of the session was filled up with the mother's "outpourings." These were related to the fact that the mother feels that there have been "three minuses" in her life, and she wants to know if they are related. All of them occurred in a two-year time span. First, she had a miscarriage at home. Then, she had a normal baby that had a viral infection—Bill said the mother expressed this "as if the child had somehow been bitten by a fly"—and died. Bill commented that the mother doesn't focus on the way that the child died: namely, the mother was feeding the child, and it aspirated in her arms. The third minus is the child with trisomy 13.
>
> Bill thought he had gotten through to the mother that there was nothing she did that caused any of the problems. The mother raised the issue of sterilization, and Bill had brought Giordano in to discuss that this was not the appropriate time to make this decision.

Bill reported that the mother was discouraged because today the baby looks good. She was hoping that it would die soon, so seeing it look healthy really discouraged her. Nancy Thomas suggested that the mother needed to do some more work dealing with this loss and the loss of her other baby.

Giordano suggested that having this mother walking around wishing her baby would die was itself a problem, and that the mother would "need" to fall apart at some time.

Berger said that having the parents actively involved could only make the situation worse. Giordano countered that their wishing the baby dead would only make them feel worse when it actually happened.

Bill closed the discussion by saying that he was not happy with the session, that the parents had gone around and around like a broken record, and that he wasn't sure that they had a better handle on things when they left.

Despite their obvious concern, all the genetic counselors do in this case is wring their hands and trade their anxieties. They neither plan to meet with the parents again nor inform the neonatologists of their worries. They are a virtual Greek chorus commenting on a tragedy which they are well-placed to observe but powerless to prevent.

The counselors are sensitive about their place in Nightingale's hierarchy of physicians. They take as one indicator of the casualness with which they are treated the difficulty they have in getting others to take their requests for help seriously. We have seen this already in their inability to coax results quickly out of pathology.[12] Another problem was getting psychiatry, another devalued medical

12. An interesting question, and one that counselors never asked, was to what degree was this a systems problem rather than an indicator of genetic counseling's status as a service. To the degree that other physicians had the same problem, it could not be an indicator of a disparagement of the worth of human genetics. The counselors never sought to find out the degree to which what they perceived as their private troubles were a public issue at Nightingale. In this case, getting results from pathology was not unique to genetic counselors. It plagued many at Nightingale Children's Center. Moreover, it is not a problem unique to Nightingale.

service at Nightingale, to respond to what the genetic counselors felt were emotional crises revealed in sessions with parents.

Bill Smith is reporting to me on a counseling session he had with Mrs. Zuverink, a woman who had a child with tuberous sclerosis. Bill felt that Mrs. Zuverink had deep-seated emotional problems. He said that Mrs. Zuverink was seeing a parish priest for counseling and at the same time getting pills from a local physician. Bill worried about the appropriateness of the treatment this woman was receiving.

During the session, he said he had been able to elicit from Mrs. Zuverink how depressed she was, how much despair she really did feel, and how she felt suicidal most of the time.

Bill then claimed that the session made him see why he didn't go into psychiatry. Bill said he was very good at getting the material on the table, but that once it was out, he didn't really know what to say, and then he felt terribly inadequate. Bill said he could always tell when he was in over his head because he got a headache.[13]

To get help for Mrs. Zuverink, Bill called the psychiatric liaison to the genetics service. Bill said that he mentioned that the woman was on pills, that she felt suicidal, and that she did not have a lot of money for treatment.

The liaison told Bill that there was not much to be done, that if the woman wanted help, she would have to pay the going rate for it.

Bill was unsettled by this. He complained to me that although he recognized the need for long-term psychiatric help, he was unable to get the psychiatrist to provide it. "I really pulled out all the stops, Bosk. I used all the tricks in my bag: I mentioned drugs, I mentioned

13. An interesting and unstudied topic is the cues that physicians use to know that they are in trouble—working beyond their "comfort zone." Here, Bill's cue is a somatic one. One general surgeon I know uses an olfactory one. He claims that whenever the operating room begins to smell like an anatomy lab, he is too fatigued to continue operating.

pills, I painted a bleak picture. And what did they do? They said when it gets bad enough, the patient will do something on her own. I don't know what you have to do around here to convince a psychiatrist that a problem is serious."

The frustration with psychiatry and the inability to refer out counseling problems further limited what genetics counselors could do for their patients. Recognizing that they were over their heads when it came to dealing with serious emotional problems, they had no one else to send those problems to. This then limited their efforts at eliciting problems and focused their attention on the service they could competently provide: accurate information about diagnosis and recurrence.

All in all, genetic counselors felt status pain whenever they were asked to mop up their colleagues' problems. They felt that they were being asked to shoulder an inappropriate amount of the hand-holding that is part and parcel of pediatric work. At the same time, they also felt status pain when they could not get others to take their requests for help seriously. The operation of routine consultation merely reinforced the low status of counselors in the hierarchy of Nightingale Children's Center.

4

BABY DOE BEFORE
REGULATIONS

When we look at workplace relations, a Hughesian perspective urges us to concentrate on routines and emergencies, with the suggestion that special care be paid to workers in the service industries. Ethnographers have discussed under this rubric the signaling patterns of ambulance drivers (Sudnow 1967), the beat-walking of skid-row policemen (Bittner 1967a, 1967b), the suicide review conferences of psychiatrists (Light 1972), the mortality and morbidity review of surgeons (Millman 1976; Bosk 1979), and the organization of infant intensive care units (Guillemin and Holmstrom 1986; Bogdan, Brown, and Foster, 1982).

For ethnographers of work, medical settings are privileged sites for studying the dramatization of routines and emergencies. Medical students are socialized to think of their behavior in terms of its quasi-divine authority: the physician decides, and the patient's fate hangs in the balance (Becker et al. 1961). For the genetic counselors, such situations are but a memory. In their current roles, they are almost never in situations where their decision determines a patient's fate. When their colleagues try to thrust more responsibility for decision making on them, they either pass it back to the physicians or the patients, both of whom the genetic counselors feel are more expert decision makers than they. Their colleagues "have decided to put on green suits"; and hence have to make decisions. The genetic counselors have declined, even on those rare occasions when they are requested to do so. Further, the patients or the parents of the patients in the genetic counselors' minds are the best decision makers because—"Well, because the odds were one in forty thousand that this could happen, and how would anyone of us know how we would respond." However, as a group they are not vocal advocates for this principle in the hospital at large.

The genetic counselors, because of their expertise, were consulted routinely when there were births with serious anomalies. On very rare occasions, these involved the genetic counselors in clinical crises for a few days. But the genetic counselors were present at these medical emergencies much more in the capacity of Rosencrantz and Guildenstern than in the role of Hamlet. As an ethnographer, as their witness, I tagged along. For the genetic counselors, emergencies involved parents whom they had counseled who wished to discontinue treatment of severely damaged neonates despite the objections of Nightingale Children's Center physicians charged with clinical responsibility. These cases all differ from the situation of the Doughertys described in the last chapter. These were all cases where parents never become convinced that they and the physicians were working toward the same goal.

This chapter describes the role that genetic counselors play in these crises of decision making as magnifiers of trouble "by supporting what we later learn are not options," and discusses the decision-making process more generally. When I made these observations, withdrawal of treatment was ethically problematic, much discussed in bioethics and pediatrics, but not yet a public and political issue.

This changed in 1981 when a Danville, Illinois couple refused to consent to surgery for duodenal atresia for their infant child born with trisomy 21. The case caught the attention of President Reagan, whose administration proposed a regulation making such refusals of treatment a violation of Public Law 92-504, which guarantees equal access to the handicapped. As a result, "Baby Doe hotlines" were established. An 800 number was posted in all infant intensive care units. Individuals could call this number and report any instances in which they observed treatment withdrawals.

Not surprisingly, the administration's proposed regulation and the establishment of the hotlines met with stiff professional resistance.[1] For a variety of reasons, the medical profession was successful at beating back the challenge to the clinical autonomy posed by Baby Doe regulations. This chapter looks at the management of Baby Doe situations before regulations to see how such situations were managed in one local network, to document one more workplace exigency for genetic counselors, and to illustrate the complexities of decision making when claims of medical autonomy collide with claims of privacy for prenatal decision making.

Even before Baby Doe hotlines, there were disagreements in neonatal intensive care units. How could it be otherwise? However, the problem is not that parents and physicians collude to kill handicapped children. Rather, the problem is just the opposite; in neonatal units hope often exceeds reason, wishes run ahead of wisdom, and the exigencies of emergency situations overwhelm sober calculations of cost and benefit in the long run. When medical care is for infants, the logical circuitry of cost-benefit reasoning disconnects, producing a perfect example of a Durkheimian cult of the individual under conditions of extreme organic and mechanical solidarity: the pediatric or neonatal intensive care unit.

In the NICUs of pediatric hospitals, the activist, individualistic ethos of American culture virtually enjoins the physician to act and the parents to wish for that action. The problem in intensive care then, is patterns of overzealous treatment, rather than neglect. What made the Baby Doe regulations such an intriguing development was that the entire drift of reports from intensive care units—whether they were autobiographical recountings of families, the reports of medical scientists in established journals, or sociological accounts of the dynamics of aggressive intervention in the NICU—indicated that the regulations, however they were modified, amended, understood, and applied, had the problem backwards (Guillemin and Holmstrom 1986; Stinson and Stinson 1979, 1983; Silverman 1981).

This chapter recounts two cases from my fieldwork experience that clearly would have been Baby Doe cases had there been such regulations at the time. In each case, parents refused initially to con-

1. For accounts of the Baby Doe regulations see Annas (1983), Guillemin and Holmstrom (1983, 1986), Murray (1985), Rhoden and Annas (1985), Robertson (1981).

sent to care for their children. In each case, physicians were divided over the parents' refusal, some supporting it as understandable and their right, some opposing it and claiming to speak as the advocates of the child. I shall use these two cases to illustrate how the philosophical and ethical dilemmas of clinical freedom, autonomy, and responsibility were framed at Nightingale.

Two Cases

The fact that genetic counselors were involved in each of these cases meant that disagreements had spilled out of the private intensive care unit into the hospital and were a source of public trouble. Because both these cases became public hospital issues, previously unacknowledged differences became visible, and there was no simple way to disentangle participants, no way to smooth over ruffled feathers. These cases are separated in time by three years. Read that way, they are a simple illustration of how little progress had been made in one major American hospital in dealing with the kinds of questions and problems that arise when the shared understanding of physicians and parents of what is in the best interests of the child breaks down. Since the last case, "ethical consultation" has become available. How that changes situations when there is a conflict of intentions between parental and medical narratives for the child (Hunter 1991) is an important topic for future exploration. My intent in providing the detail I do in describing these cases is to give a sense of a "same-old, used-to-be" to describe the pediatrics hospital before "ethics" had a widespread presence at the bedside.

One last prefatory note: That the cases are separated by three years means that the depth of my access to data and my understanding of that data was different. When the first case arose, I was literally a few days in the field. It was my first attendance at rounds. I was unknown to many and trusted by few of the people in the setting. The second case became an issue at the end of my three years in the setting. By this time, more than a little trust had been built up. This case I was able to observe quite closely. I was quite literally dragged along into all negotiations by Palmer as "someone who could provide us some advice on what we are doing." The clear implication of this inclusion was that my advice was in the service, the thrall really, of Palmer's objectives. I was asked to be a witness, and also not to limit myself to witnessing alone. If I could provide some advice on how to avoid a disaster, in either human or public-relations terms, I should feel free to do so.

CASE 1: THE BABY

Case 1 is not so much a case as a discussion that occurred in clinical genetics rounds, the weekly meeting of pediatricians, social workers, nurses, and lab technicians who are involved in the ongoing work of the genetic counseling team. Dr. Bill Smith presented the case. He began by stating that for reasons "that would become clear," he neither wanted to bring the child down for the group (which numbered around thirty) to see, nor did he want the group to visit the bedside. That much said, he began to present the baby's history. He reported that he first saw the baby at ten hours of age. (Interestingly, in this case the baby was always referred to as *the baby* and never as *Baby Girl Smith* or even *the baby girl.*) The baby, he reported, had been born with multiple birth defects. The child was born without three limbs, without a jaw, with fusion of lip and palate, and with splenic-gonadal fusion. He continued his reporting: There was no known history of consanguinity in the family, nor was there any history of drug intake during pregnancy. Neurologically, the child was as alert as a neonate should be. Given this clinical picture, he concluded that a diagnosis of one of the mandibular syndromes with limb hypogenesis best fit the baby. These, he informed the group, were all mostly sporadic. At this point Dr. Smith had completed the normal presentation of a case during genetic rounds: he had described the physical findings, identified the syndrome associated with those findings, and provided a recurrence risk.

At this point, the normal order of rounds would have been to discuss Dr. Smith's diagnosis—evaluate its adequacy—or if there were no questions, move on to the next case. But in this case, something else happened.[2] Dr. Smith continued his narrative. He said, "I

2. There is a little retrospective judgment here. I could not, at the time (this being a first viewing of rounds), have known how this case was not typical or normal.

don't know if this is the place to bring it up, but we've been agonizing over it for days now. The child has severe defects. The parents have asked for no surgical procedures. The surgeons are convinced this is a salvageable child, [who] has no life-threatening problems and will live with minor surgery. The parents plainly do not want any surgery."

Dr. Berger, chief of the genetics unit, was the first to speak after Smith had laid the doctors' dilemma on the table. He said, "We know how the Spartans felt about such babies. We are dealing here with a severely damaged child. It is hard to get the family to accept what is an impossible situation. We have to take a very hard, philosophical approach. This is a little like the thalidomide babies."

The baby's pediatrician, Dr. Abbott, refocused the discussion on the parents' rejection of the child and their resistance to surgical intervention: "The parents do not want this child treated. They do not want the child to go home. They have voiced this over and over again."

Berger here reminds the group that this is a statement which cannot be tolerated. "But obviously some future has to be faced. Not in one year. Not in two years. But now."

At this point, a physician whose name I had not yet learned, asked the question which until then had not been asked directly: "What if the family absolutely refuses surgery?"[3]

The question invited speculation. This baby, these parents. These times (the early years of the Carter administration). This surgeon. Those lawyers. This hospital administration. With so much variation, each new case has only weak precedents. Dr. Berger, official leader of the group, took a stab at answering the question: "Well, we have to know what is the position of the hospital and what is the position of the parents in making this decision. In making these decisions, the courts have in the past made a plan for the child. Of course, it's also possible in the current climate that the courts

3. Remember this is my first day in this setting. I did not know who was who. I was phenomenologically overloaded. I had heard that physicians discussed such things, but I had never heard such a discussion. It was hard enough to grasp what was being said, let alone record who was saying what. Sometimes, the trickiest bit of ethnographic work is the first part: the getting straight of who said what to whom.

would let the child die.[4] But such a course would be hard. I gather from the consultants that the plastic surgeons think they can do something for the child, and rehabilitation thinks they can do something for the child."

Realizing that the drift of this logic is into the surgical suite, Dr. Eggleston attacks a basic underlying premise of Berger's argument: the analogy to thalidomide babies. "Yes, but this is not like the thalidomide babies. Here we need an intervention. This is different. You have to make a positive decision to undertake surgery."

As far as Berger is concerned, *plus ça change, plus c'est la même chose:* "But it is only minor surgery. A conservative approach would be to intervene, because this is a rehabilitable child."

At this point, Smith reenters the conversation with the observation that "socially, the parents want to abandon the child." Berger points out to him the distance between the desiring and the doing: "I don't know how easy it is for parents to abandon children."[5]

The questioner who opened up this whole sequence by asking, What if the parents absolutely refused? now complicates his own hypothetical question: "What would we do if the parents were Seventh-Day Adventists?" Smith, perhaps uneasy about all of this speculation, reports another item of the parents' behavior: "The parents have asked to have the child killed." This is a request that Berger takes at face value. "That's a shock reaction." The doctors' dilemma won't go away: What if they absolutely refuse? The original framer of this hypothetical question projects it into the future: "What if they took the child home and it died? What if we did nothing? Could they be prosecuted?"[6]

4. Berger's estimate of the current climate has only grown more accurate. At any rate, invocations of the "current climate" are extemporaneous judgment. There is a recurrent frustration in writing about the "current climate" in applied clinical genetics: the climate changes quickly; the publication process for any report on the current climate is much slower.

5. According to a considerable historical literature, it may not be so difficult for parents to abandon children as Berger suggests. Certainly, evidence of child abandonment is not absent in contemporary American society. To be fair, the normative response appears to be the opposite: parents assume responsibility for less-than-perfect newborns.

6. The questioner might have asked about his own legal liability here as well: Is silence consent? And if in all this there is a felony and felons, are there not also ac-

Smith fields this question with a discussion of what the drill is for today, not tomorrow: "This is all becoming a question of hospital policy." He then states his understanding of that policy: "We are not going to starve this child. If it arrests, we are not going to resuscitate." This is not a policy nor a plan that satisfies Berger. He grumbles: "That's wishing away a bad situation, and it's not just going to go away. The child is not going to die."

Berger's remark seems to generate yet another hypothetical question: "If the state intervenes and if the child undergoes surgery, then who is financially responsible?" The normally pragmatic Berger fails to answer this question and responds with a Panglossian piety: "These are extreme situations which we are beginning to face everyday; whose financial problem is the child? This is such a rare situation. It's a chance event. Why should we victimize the parents and tell them to dedicate their lives because of a random event. If society decides that these children should be saved, then let society take care of them. And let us let the parents come to some moral and spiritual resolution of this situation themselves."

Berger has a certain sympathy for Smith's immediate problems. But he reminds him and the assembled group that the parents should not be crushed because the physicians found themselves squeezed between the rock of what a physician's sense of responsibility obligated him or her to do and the hard place of the society's lack of resources for dealing with the chronically handicapped: "Well, we can't treat these parents like they are victims of the Inquisition. Who knows how any of us would react? We can't force people either to cope or not to cope with such extreme situations."

At this point, the physician who originally objected to the thalidomide analogy reinvokes it: "There's always the danger of brainwashing the parents. You're always citing the exceptions, the children, the thalidomide children who did well."

Berger agrees: "Yes, we also have this with myelomeningocele, where two-thirds are retarded. Yet we are always talking about the one-third that does well. And now society is getting more and more

---

cessories? The boundaries in these matters, being set by prosecutorial creativity, are difficult to trace with precision.

into the act, which is very much different than saying, 'Here's your baby, go find a quiet cliff and deal with it.'"

Smith at this point adds an encouraging note: "Well, we are evolving solutions to these problems. But they [the parents] are trying to make the baby disappear. We're trying to keep it alive." At this point, Berger closed discussion of the case with the pronouncement: "Well, we can't make an ultimate projection of what the parents will do or how the baby will do in the long run."

Let me note that the case had the following resolution. Surgery was planned despite the parents' objections. However, as this was all happening, the infant developed a breathing problem and died. Berger was wrong; some bad situations do disappear. Three years later, the parents gave birth to a healthy infant.

Time Passes

It is three years later. All the contextual variables in which clinical decisions are made have changed. The field of applied human genetics has advanced technically. Changes are, of course, too numerous to detail here and still discuss the process of decision making when parents challenge physicians; nevertheless, some deserve mention. Operationally, the most important is that the status of amniocentesis has changed from that of a procedure that is assumed safe, but not definitively known to be so, to one whose safety has been documented by the Canadian, United States, and United Kingdom registry studies. Amniocentesis is now a clinical routine of obstetrics. Further advances in the technology of cytogenetics have made it possible to identify genetic abnormalities through increasingly subtle "markers." At the same time, technical progress in the field of neonatal intensive care has made it possible to salvage babies of lower and lower birth weights. The American public has been kept aware of such advances and their downside risks through local television media, local newspapers, and a variety of national magazines, including *Consumer Reports, Atlantic,* and *Time.*

At a local level, both the genetic counseling group and the facilities for neonatal intensive care have evolved. Most obviously, its members, in Schutz's memorable phrase, "have grown older together" (1971, 220). Over three years, operating rules of thumb, tacit understandings, and informal norms for handling work have been in constant flux because of changes in membership.[7] Twice now, clinic coordinators have come and gone. A social worker or genetics associate, the clinic coordinator is a key figure in organizing the work of the genetics group. More significantly, Berger, the leader and academic patron of the younger physicians who are genetic counselors, has left. His replacement, Dr. Palmer, is an unknown quantity. His investment in the "special mission" of genetic counseling is suspect. However, as chair of the Pediatrics Department, his political authority in the hospital is firmly established. Careers are at stake in personnel changes such as this; it was a highly stressful time for the genetic counselors. Brooding about the future had become a very popular collective activity.

Things have not been all that calm in either the newborn nursery or the neonatal intensive care unit either. Nurses in the newborn nursery have taken issue on several occasions with physicians' decisions both to attempt or to refrain from attempting salvage of compromised neonates. After much wrangling, an official policy has been outlined detailing the broad criteria on which judgments are based.

Despite this effort, a lack of clarity still remains about the process of making judgments: who is involved, with what authority, and with what dispute-resolution mechanisms are all areas of continuing uncertainty. Meanwhile, intensive care has become one of the areas where the "action" is in pediatrics. The nurses view themselves as an elite corps with special skills, disposition, and courage. The field also has a charisma and ethos for physicians similar to what Fox and Swazey describe for cardiac surgeons (1974). As Guillemin and Holmstrom document so well, in the world of pediatric intensive care, physicians and nurses casually wear their "courage to fail" ethos on the sleeves of their scrub suits.

Moreover, what Berger referred to as the "current climate" when speculating about what actions the courts might take if the parents absolutely refused surgery has changed. First, a significant right-

7. Numerous as these changes are, flux is perhaps the normal standard of things in American teaching hospitals, what with regular rotations, academic leave, and the normal mobility that is part of a career.

to-life group has moved politically from the fringe to the main-stream—to breakfast at prayer meetings with a newly elected president. These groups have grown more militant and aggressive in their protection of fetal and neonatal "rights." All of the physicians at the pediatric hospital were well aware of the potential politicization of any decision not to treat, and the attendant media spectacle that could result. How this constrained their thinking about cases is difficult to gauge precisely; that it did so is undeniable.

Finally, the fieldworker has changed as well. I took in the first case described here with the phenomenological wonder of a child. The second I took in with a sense of phenomenological fatigue, a weariness from seeing all too many of what the genetic counselors refer to as "God's mistakes." In fact at the time of the second case, I had officially withdrawn from the field, ostensibly to begin writing up my data. However, the impending birth of my first child made it unbearable to see, on a routine basis, so many parents whose desires for a "perfect" baby had been disappointed at the start. I was called back both by Smith and by Palmer, each of whom for reasons of their own wanted a sounding board to share their thoughts, feelings, and frustrations as the case unfolded. Smith and Palmer had been generous with themselves as informants; I owed them much, and I could not easily refuse their request to help out by observing a case that they described as "one I would be interested in."[8] I returned to the field, but I took notebook in hand with much reluctance.

To provide some comparability between the discussions of the two cases, I shall, as with the first case, report only on one conference, despite the fact that I was privy to much more. The conference was called after the contest over clinical autonomy was resolved, and its purpose was to review that resolution.

CASE 2: BABY BOY FLANNERY

Baby Boy Flannery had been born seven days previously with trisomy 21 and duodenal atresia (a stricture in the intestine that

8. Ethnographers have not, as a rule, spent enough time thinking about how our subjects produce data for us on the basis of their judgments of what we might find interesting; how they place us "on call" for the things they think we want to see.

makes normal feeding impossible). At the time that the neonatologist explained the treatment options to the father, he included in his presentation the right to refuse surgery. The father of the child (the mother at this time was not yet informed of the child's problems) chose to exercise this option. This decision was unacceptable to the nursing staff of the newborn nursery—they refused to carry it out. For them, not treating in this instance was not a branch of the decision tree. Operationally, the nurses on staff had the organized authority to call the question. As a group, they rejected not treating as an option. The neonatologists then negotiated an agreement late on a Friday afternoon to assume custody of the baby, arrange for its transfer to Nightingale which is affiliated with the newborn nursery, repair its stomach, and then place it up for adoption.

First thing Monday morning, Friday's agreement proved unworkable. No mechanisms existed, to the satisfaction of all parties for the parents quickly and definitively to relinquish custody, for the courts to authorize repair, for the surgeons to repair, and for the child to secure "an alternative parental environment."[9] Nightingale Children's Center refused to accept transfer of the child without a surgical consent. Tuesday passed trying to arrange transfer of the child to another hospital that would agree to nonrepair. No hospital could be found. By this time, a third party ready to press for the child's right to life in court had materialized. On Wednesday, the parents agreed to the transfer. On Thursday, the surgery was done. Friday was conference day.

I was informed of the conference about two hours before it was to begin, by Bill Smith. I asked Smith what the hurry was. He told me that he had objected strongly to the conference: "It's appropriate to have a conference when the dust has settled, but not now, you know what I mean? Emotionally and scientifically, what good can it do now? People are too involved."[10] He pointed out that, as a rule,

9. The quotation marks here indicate not a naive usage at the time, but a relabeling years later by me of this last question, which was the place where understanding broke down.

10. Ethnographers often criticize documentary journalism for "putting into words" subjects' private thoughts. We ethnographers don't do that sort of thing, of course. But here I report a "snatch" from a private phone conversation. What kind of person behaves this way? Don't accurate reports from the backstage inevitably vio-

death and dying conferences were held two weeks after the event, and that gave people a little time to cool out. He said that he was "frightened" about what could come out of a conference. Smith told me that, "knowing no good" could come of this conference, he had tried to block the neonatology fellow from scheduling it. The fellow, whom he described as a stubborn type, dug in his heels and would not reschedule the conference. Smith went over his head and called one of the attendings in neonatology. From him he learned that the entire group of neonatologists wanted the conference and wanted it now. As a group, they had all supported offering the nontreatment option to the parents. They felt "sandbagged" by the administration. The group was "angry, very angry" and, "short of quitting," did not know what to do. The neonatologists felt that they were "being told how to practice medicine and that they had been blocked from a legitimate treatment option."

It's worth noting that at the time (1981), the neonatologists had every reason in the world to believe that they had indeed been sandbagged. It's also worth noting that times have changed. A new norm has emerged. Today the neonatologists are much less likely to support the parents. The parents, faced with in-hospital ethical help, are less likely to push the point. But consensus reached is not always consensus sustained. Scarce resources, the need to constrain medical cost, less collective generosity for the chromosomally different—all threaten the current ethical consensus. One never knows until cases make new problems. But back then, the physicians were sandbagged, and the nurses were right. Operationally, not treating was not part of the decision tree at Nightingale.

The conference, which was scheduled for 1:00 P.M., started a mere ten minutes later, a remarkable display of punctuality for such an ad hoc meeting. There were twenty-seven people in attendance: representatives of neonatology, genetics, surgery, and social services, as well as several "interested" members of the hospital community who had heard about the case. Dr. Mackrides—head of the Newborn Nursery—sat on the left front side of the table; Dr. Pal-

---

late some sort of privacy? And, more gloomy still, doesn't the violation of privacy by individual ethnographic actions weaken privacy as a collective ideal?

mer, at the right. Whether ominously or innocently, no one took that place at the head of the table. Dr. Mackrides began the conference. She directed everybody's attention to a handout detailing what happened when, gave a brief oral summary of the case, announced the purpose of the meeting as being "to discuss what happened," and turned the floor over to Dr. Palmer.

Dr. Palmer began: "This is an instructive case, just as all cases should be instructive to physicians. The first thing we need to do is recognize the physician's responsibility in cases of this sort. The first responsibility of the physician is to give an expert explanation of Down's syndrome, trisomy 21, and its obvious association with the vomiting in this case. This was done right from the beginning, since Dr. Smith had met with the family [the father] for three hours on Friday, the day the child was born. What is known in this case is that the child has a relatively easily correctable defect, that it is a viable child without heart disease but with mongolism. Rather than to inject our own values into the case, our responsibility is to present every reasonable treatment option. In this case we learned what our reasonable options are; we also learned what the nonviable options are. For twenty-four to forty-eight hours, we had all thought we would be able to assume custody of the child. The next time this happens—and the next time will probably be next week, since these things happen in twos and threes—well, we'll know that option is not present."[11]

There was then some discussion in which various members of the hospital staff involved with the case all expressed their surprise at finding out that the transfer of custody was legally complicated. One member of the audience was incredulous. He asked, "How does this case differ from guardianship? Hospitals assume guardianship all the time. How is this different from going to the courts and getting an order?"

Mackrides does not so much answer this question as frame all the

11. Palmer's reference here to things happening in cascades ("twos and threes") reflects a widespread folk-belief among physicians that rare events cluster in time in ways that defy mere statistical probability. Certainly, the general surgeons I have studied (Bosk 1979) shared this belief. I suppose it could be empirically tested. But if the belief was not verified, was shown to be mere "occupational superstition," it would not matter much. The workgroup in the hospital is not without its genuine need for some magical thinking.

hospital's actions as being guided by the goal of providing the parents support. She says, "In our attempts to support the parents, we did not want to obtain a court order. We felt that that would be violating the rights, the beliefs, the whatever-you-have, of the parents. We decided not to take the case to court, but to try and support them."

Dr. Palmer places this support in the larger context of alternative scenarios the physicians might have had to face in this case. "I want to back up and talk about the options. The first is to tell the parents what mongolism is and means, to say that the child has no heart lesion but, with gastrointestinal surgery, will be a normal Down's syndrome child, and then have the parents say, 'This is a child, this is our child, and this is one we want to take home. We want the child to be repaired.' Obviously this did not happen in this case. That brings us to option two. Here the parents say, 'We want the child to have normal surgery and care, and we will reserve the decision about the child's ultimate disposition. We will all work together to make long-run decisions in the future.' This option was also rejected in this case. The parents then have option three—they can say, 'We have decided we do not want the child to live. We feel in our hearts that we cannot let this child come into our home. We cannot let this child live.' If the parents choose this option, as was the case here, then there are two branching options that have to be considered: Whether this will happen in this institution, or whether the child will go elsewhere. It is this hospital's policy not to carry out neglect both for legal reasons and because of the institution's philosophy. This leaves parents the option of taking the child home to die. Frankly, I would not have mentioned to the parents the option of refusing surgery. It confused the parents, and we all did not appreciate the legal aspects of taking the child home. The parents could be slapped with a neglect or a murder suit by the prosecutors. The way this case evolved, the parents—we all—had to be educated to their real options. At any time, the institution could have said, 'We'll go to the courts.' But we wanted to help the parents to come to the right decision, and a court order would have created more problems than it would have solved. At one time, the parents' lawyer and the hospital's lawyer went to the courts to gather information privately. Now I wasn't a party to those dicussions, but the parents must have found they had no good option, because they decided to sign for surgery."

Dr. Farley, a pediatrician interested in medical ethics, felt Palmer's presentation narrowed the parents' options unreasonably. "I think the parents got bad advice if they were told that they didn't have the right to refuse treatment. The trend in this country in the courts so far has been to maximize the patient's right to refuse care. No state has gone against this trend. The most recent case which has a bearing here—the New Jersey Supreme Court ruling in the Quinlan case—sees this decision as a private matter between the family and the physicians. As one looks over twenty years of legal precedent, the right to maximize refusal seems to be fairly well established. The option to refuse treatment is real in many states, including a neighboring one. As far as I am concerned the rights of the child and of the parents have been abrogated in this case."

Palmer responded, "Let's assume that what you say is correct—and I'm not willing to grant that—our institutional policy is not to support neglect. We will support parents in their decision making. I am familiar with a case where the parents took the child home, and it died later. The parents could go somewhere else. Either way, if you go either way, you have to be very certain in this state, in this country, of the legal ramifications—be sure you know what is going to happen to you. I am not a lawyer. I am not a judge. I am not God. Both the parents and I have to be sure no prosecutor is going to bring charges."

Dr. Mackrides here tried to move the discussion from hypothetical to empirical matters. "If the parents had refused, the hospital was determined, if it did not get permission within a certain time, to get a court order. This is not a personal theory; this was going to happen."

Farley here points out that there is a difference between trying to obtain a court order and actually having one. "But the court could have said no. This is a matter of privacy. It is between the families and physicians to agree on a course of action. In fact, it is hard to imagine the courts countermanding the parents' decision to refuse."

There is one weakness in Farley's hypothetical point; it is an empirical one, and Palmer is quick to point it out. "If that is the case," he wanted to know, "why did they go to court on Wednesday and come away signing for the operation."

Farley is undeterred. He maintains, with a correctness more fitting to law review articles than to everyday life, that "the trend in the law is to back away from such matters and call them private."

As this debate on legal theory wound down, Dr. Mackrides added a new piece of information. "I should mention here that a member of a child-advocate group called me to get information on the child in order to get an injunction to forbid the parents from signing the child out against medical advice. It was a matter of timing. If the parents had signed out AMA, an agency was going to get an injunction that would have tried to force the parents to consent to surgery." Palmer pointed out that this was an example of a point he had been trying to make, that the parents were bound to be put under lots of pressure.

Dr. Kraft, a neonatologist, asked, "What finally turned the parents around?"

Palmer answered, "I wish I knew."

Here the surgeon who performed the surgery added a pious homily: "May I suggest that the case was turned around because the parents realized that we were—that the doctors in this case realized that it was not just a child but a family that needed help—that we came *to* but not *at* the parents." He added that the family was now considering taking the child home.

Dr. Mackrides had some difficulty with this description. "That is a very idealistic picture. I think what happened was that they exhausted all other possibilities. My perception is that at one point they were asking what is worse, the publicity from signing or not signing. They repeatedly talked about the publicity, the newspapers, the intrusion on their private lives. It wasn't an idealistic move. Right now they are exploring adoption agencies."

At this point, someone asked, "What if they had refused?"

Palmer responded, "That is a reasonable question. I had decided if they wanted to sign out AMA, that we would allow them to do so. Any hospital has to allow this. I cannot answer what I would have done if they had signed out—if I had an obligation to report neglect, to seek an injunction, to file a CY 147 [a report of suspected child abuse]. I think personally I would not have sought an injunction, but as to whether the hospital would have, I do not know." For Palmer, who is chairman of pediatrics of the hospital, this distinction between what he would do and what the hospital would do is an extreme equivocation or an act of public discretion. What is interesting is what is not said: what the hospital would have done. And surely as a the doer of hospital action, Palmer had at least a theory about that. His "personal" position is clear. His official, "public" policy is not articulated.[12]

Someone points out, "But there was a third party ready to seek an injunction."

Palmer answers, "There is always a third party in this kind of institution."

At this point, a short discussion of adoption policy and lots of side involvement mark the meeting. The discussion is put on course by a neonatology fellow who asks, "What about the charge that the parents were badgered, that they were in a grief reaction, and that they couldn't make up their minds. Why didn't we use hyperal solution to hydrate the baby until the parents got over the initial shock?"

Mackrides, Palmer, and the surgeon all assured the questioner that this was exactly what happened. Following this, Farley objected that all the effort in this case had been toward coercing consent and that nontreatment was never realistically considered. Palmer stated that no one in the hospital had threatened the parents with legal action, but that they themselves bowed before the legal threat nontreatment represented.

Mackrides added, "A major side of this case hasn't been discussed. When the parents first decided not to treat, prior to their attempts to relinquish custody, I had agreed with the parents' decision not to support it. I went to the nurses to say that this is the situation. Here is the baby, we are not going to support it. I had a nursing revolt on my hands. My young nurses looking at this healthy baby couldn't carry out this decision. They thought this was a place to maintain life. The same sentiment emerged among medical students, house officers, and fellows. The question I have is

12. Because Palmer speaks for himself, no one speaks for the hospital; a curious omission.

how to carry out a decision that involves such grief and pain to my staff."

Palmer said that he had been through this once or twice before and that "inevitably the surgery gets done. If the physicians agree to support the parents, the administration doesn't. If administration is supportive, then the nurses aren't. And if the nurses support the parents, and they inevitably do not, then there are outside threats. The best thing to do is to defuse the situation as quickly and quietly as possible."

One neonatologist stated, "Then one of the things we have learned is not doing anything is not an option."

Farley objected that it was important that it remain an option.

Palmer responded, "No, logically, it is not an option. Because here you are using duodenal atresia as a method of euthanasia. I want to sort that out. We can't use one condition as a reason for euthanasia because of another condition, mongolism."

This would have seemed to end the discussion, but someone asked if the parents had to be told before the surgery that the child had trisomy 21. A long discussion on truth-telling and its pros and cons followed. Once this discussion ended, Dr. Mackrides began to wrap up the conference. "No one can deny that it is a difficult problem. I have calculated that excluding today's conference, 386 man-hours have gone to resolving it. Perhaps Dr. Palmer would like to make a few concluding remarks."

Palmer states, "This case has been an important learning experience. What is important is that now we know what the real options are. What caused such problems here is that we held out to the parents an option that didn't exist. In the future, we must avoid this. We must judge each case on its own merits with respect for the dignity of the persons involved. We must recognize that there are at least three patients." But there is a contradiction here, for if all trisomy 21 children will be operated on, if that is the general rule, then there is no reason to look at each case on its merits.

This speech closed the conference. As I left the room, Palmer came over to me. He asked me what I thought. I shrugged my shoulders. He said, "If this is what goes on at Mecca, I would hate to see how these things are handled in the boondocks."

TIME STOPS

The two cases which I have presented so far have been displayed in greater detail than is normal in ethnographic analysis. In the conventional presentation of this type of firsthand observational data, field examples are usually pressed into service to underline particular points. My warrant for forgoing the normal procedure is provided by Hauerwaus, who suggests that ethical analysis dispense with the question, What should we do? and concern itself instead with How do we know we are describing the situation correctly? Hauerwaus goes on to say, "Unlike mud puddles, situations are not something that we simply fall into. Situations and the decisions we make about them are what they are because of the presumptions we hold and how we have come to see them" (1977). What I have attempted to do in the case presentation is describe the situations, decisions, and presumptions that make decision-making autonomy in medicine so problematic. Such a description does not, of course, speak for itself. In this section, I turn to an analysis and interpretation of the situations, decisions, and presumptions that governed decision-making in the two Baby Doe analogues presented above.

Before doing so, let me add a gratuitous editorial comment or two, so that the reader can better gauge my own biases. First, although the parents' desire for nontreatment is similar in the two cases, each presents to the pediatricians involved very different questions. Had I been required to act rather than just observe, my response to each case would have been very different. In the first case, I would have had no problems with nontreatment. The magnitude of the child's problems, the potential quality of life, the parents' response—all of these made intervention appear less than noble to me. In addition, I never escaped the feeling that an overly optimistic picture of the child's future was being projected by the surgeons and the physicians in rehabilitation medicine—this feeling was confirmed by the child's demise. But there was no necessity to this. Save for a "breathing problem," a miracle might have been manufactured.

With the second case, like Palmer, like the parents as the situation unfolded, I am extremely uncomfortable using duodenal atresia as a pretext for euthanasia of children with trisomy 21. But, like Farley,

I am troubled by the constriction of choices. The hospital's mode of resolving the problem unsettled me. I am not sure that the parents hadn't become the victims to the Inquisition that the recently departed Berger had warned about in the first case.

Collective vs. Individual Responsibility

For me, as a sociologist, the most striking feature of the way each of the two cases is defined is this: No single physician claims decision-making authority in either case. Health care in America is not yet socialized; yet it certainly seems that, at least in this hospital, responsibility for patients has been.This jointly held responsibility explains why conflicts over nontreatment were so difficult to resolve. In complex bureaucratic settings such as hospitals, with their delimited zones of formal authority, patients move in and out of different administrative classifications, confusing who is in charge. The discourse by the physicians does not stress individual responsibility. Rather it frames the question collectively: "What should *we* as a medical staff do?" This framing recognizes how often responsibility is transferred either temporarily to a colleague on call or, more permanently, to those outside the NICU. Collective rather than individual responsibility maximizes the opportunity for a group consensus to operate, but it maximizes as well the potential for disagreement and, absent mechanisms for resolving such discord, it maximizes the opportunities for decision-making paralysis.

There are, it should go without saying, some structural features related to the organization of care which reinforce this pattern of collective decision making. First, the patients are neonates. By definition, there is no long-standing relationship with a family on which to draw in evaluating treatment options. The therapeutic relationship here is among strangers.[13] Second, the staffing patterns of the NICU encourage collective responsibility. Attendings are on for a week, rotate off for two, and then are back on. When on, attendings have total responsibility; when off, only so much as they

13. Rosenberg (1987) pointed out that relationships among strangers are a feature of hospitalized care more generally. In the ICU setting, the nature of being a stranger is amplified.

wish to assume. As a result, attendings know that they will have to live with a certain number of collegial decisions that they night have handled otherwise and vice versa.

In addition, most of the problematic cases fall outside the boundaries of what might be called normal intensive care. These are neonates with multisystem problems. Thus, to the team of intensive care physicians are added all the consultants that inhabit modern research centers. In cases of disagreement, these physicians not only have to consider the well-being of the individual patient, they need to consider their future work relations with one another. In cases where parents disagree with physicians, and physicians disagree with one another, a recurrent question is, "How are the claims of these parents whom I deal with but once matched against the claims of colleagues I need to work with day in and day out."

There are a number of dangers inherent in defining the clinical responsibility as collective. The first is, of course, that although decision making involves hordes of physicians, it is not collective in any deeper sense which reflects a communal consensus, which echoes a shared normative order. Rather, it might just as well be the case that when all the physicians gather together in one room, colleagues bow to those physicians involved with the strongest feelings about what should be done. In the two cases presented above, the pediatric surgeon consulted was also a born-again Christian with very strong feelings about each child's right to life. Here the confluence of personal beliefs and professional capacity operates to nullify parental choice.

In a context that looks like open debate, something else operates. That something else is very close to the tendency to view clinical autonomy in *absolute* terms and to brand any infringement of it as anathema. From such a viewpoint, peer review of medical care, technology assessment, cost-benefit approaches to alternative therapeutic regimes, consulting with ethics committees, and so on are unacceptable and are therefore resisted. Absolute views of clinical freedom likewise discount patient wishes and quality-of-life arguments. The general point is that conceptions of collective responsibility with special structures and processes do not of themselves guarantee enlightened decision making. Especially when inside the collective forum, some believe that no limits may sensibly be placed on the physician's duty to save a life. In this ethos it is playing God to limit the physician, while aggressive treatment is a human thing to do. That the terms of the debate might be skewed is rarely, if ever the focus of the debate.

So seen, collective responsibility in some ways reduces each decision maker's stake in the outcome. This allows those without some special interest to leave the field to those with ideological axes to grind. Collective rituals of decision sharing can become ways in which responsibility is abrogated as well as embraced. As a result, the genetic counselors, whatever their misgivings about their colleagues' actions, collude with those colleagues. They act less as mediators of conflict and more as facilitators for treatments that they do not necessarily approve. When parents do not dig in their heels, little conflict is generated. However, when parents resist, the kinds of tensions these cases illustrate proliferate. Genetic counselors, however, (in the language of the housestaff) are not "players" in resolving this trouble. Their position is clear; their value-neutrality and commitment to client autonomy lead them to support parents. Yet their actions do not reinforce their sentiments. Their deference to "green-suited claims to authority" renders them unable even to articulate these sentiments.

If the questions of others do not constrain aggressive NICU intervention, neither does the allocation of the costs of mistakes and misjudgments. None of the key medical decision makers have to live with any of the consequences of their decisions. There are no economic costs that fall upon providers from salvaging infants that are better left unsalvaged. Because in the American system there is no fixed sum allocated for health-care, there is no pressure on any individual physicians to consider the costs of a treatment, or the resource implications of salvaging a particular child, or even what it might mean to the emotional life of the family. This is not to say that individual physicians never consider these issues, but that there is very little incentive for them to do so. This reinforces whatever tendencies exist to divorce clinical action from individual responsibility. In the first case, had the child lived, the physicians involved were in a position to congratulate themselves, and they would have been shielded to a large degree from any of the negative features of the salvage. As much as the genetic counselors may have felt it was wrong "to victimize the parents and force the parents to dedicate their lives to a random event," they seemed, if not quite willing to allow that to happen, powerless to stop it. Moreover, had it happened, all of the actors debating what to do would have had limited long-term involvement with the family. This allows the freedom to intervene, whether it is individual or collective, to operate without a commensurate sense of responsibility for consequences.

Public vs. Private

The second layer of complexity in these cases rests on whether they are defined as public or private issues. In the first case we see in Berger's comments about the tendency of society to get involved the realization that old ways are changing. Three years later this change is complete, at least in the minds of medical personnel. A generalized fear of third parties dominates discussion of the second case. Only marginally does concern about what they should do guide the doctors' talk about the case. Rather, there is a preoccupation with what others will do if they pursue this or that course of action. Significantly, this concern is grounded in reality, the dubious direct interest of others in the case notwithstanding. For example, in Danville, Illinois, the aftermath of a "do not feed" order involving newborn Siamese twins illustrates just how decisive third parties can be (Robertson 1981). Nurses in the hospital disobeyed the order and secretly fed the twins. The Illinois Department of Children and Family Services was given an anonymous tip that the children were ordered to be starved to death. Armed with custody and transfer orders, the department and state's attorney moved to protect the lives of the twins. Charges of attempted murder (and thirteen other lesser offenses) were brought against the parents and physicians on the basis of complicity in the "do not feed" order.

In the more recently publicized Baby Jane Doe case, a Vermont lawyer and right-to-life advocate filed briefs to overturn a Long Island couple's refusal to consent to surgery for their severely damaged newborn.[14] What goes on in the doctor-patient rela-

---

14. One outcome of the second Baby Doe case was to limit the judicial standing of such distant third parties.

tionship is clearly not private and confidential in any ordinary sense. There appears to exist a rather wide audience of interested bystanders ready to act if the clinical autonomy of doctor and/or patient strays too widely from some unspecified rule about what is just and moral. This problem is, of course, exacerbated in an American context, where care is framed in a rhetoric of individual rights and entitlements rather than in a rhetoric of balancing collective needs.

Further, the difficulties of exercising autonomy in an intensive care setting are amplified by a design feature of the environment. As most are well aware, the typical intensive care unit is one of several large open rooms. Their design makes it possible to wheel in whatever supportive equipment is necessary to support life and to permit monitoring of patients from a single vantage point. All action is public: it takes place in the open in full view of the entire medical and nursing staff, as well as visitors to the unit. Ethics of the practice aside, it is physically impossible to leave infants to the side to die; there is no such place out of the view of others.

Although the treatment of neonates at the margin of viability is a public issue, it has a private dimension as well. As Guillemin an Holmstrom point out, "almost all American babies are hospital born, and, if critically ill, are transported to intensive care within a closed bureaucratic system managed by like-minded hospital personnel. The transfer of an infant from a community hospital to a central hospital, or from an obstetric division to the NICU in the same hospital, avoids critical outside judgment. The captive-clientele nature of critically ill newborns referred to intensive care reduces the possibility of conflict about referral, and consequently, the chances of legal dispute" (1983, 94). Furthermore, intensive care is regionalized in the American system. As a result, transport often removes parents from an effective decision-making role. The complexity and immediacy of much of the decision making regarding critically ill newborns also makes such activity a private medical matter, further reducing the parents' involvement.

There are two sides to the public and private nature of decision making in intensive care. By and large, the majority of cases become private decisions of the medical staff. In those rare cases where parents object to medical action, or physicians and parents agree to cease salvage efforts, the public nature of the decision is likely to come into play. This issue is framed in terms of the infant's rights and the threat that nontreatment poses not just to this infant, but to the class of all such infants. In the American context, there are really quite limited opportunities for withholding treatment from infants. The pressure in the American context is for treatment. Needless to say, automatic treatment is hardly a careful balancing of interests. In this light, the two cases presented above are interesting for what they reveal about how physicians feel constrained by forces well outside their control.

Professional vs. Personal Considerations

The third and last aspect of the cases under discussion that warrants discussion is the types of rationales which support action. Here we find the greatest divergence between medical and lay decision makers. It is a sociological commonplace to claim that medical authority in particular and professional authority in general rests on mastery of a formal body of theoretic knowledge. Physicians in Nightingale's intensive care units see their patients in terms of malfunctioning systems and what is needed to correct them. Talk about patients at rounds is organized by a ten-point checklist, or systems review. Residents refer to the discussion of cases at rounds as "going down the numbers." There is no irony here, the talk about patients in rounds is almost entirely talk about numbers. Discussion of family variables is rare enough to prompt a request to return to the topic (Frader and Bosk 1981). Progress is thought of in numeric terms: Are today's numbers better than yesterday's? All of this technical talk may be necessary if sick neonates are to be cared for properly. It is the essence of professional mastery. It is also a radical decontextualization of the patient as a person.

Physicians as professionals think about patients in one other set of professional terms: Physicians have also come to speculate about the legal bearing of their actions. Both cases presented in this chapter contain a great deal of hypothetical legal thinking. This is the most common form of ethical discourse that one finds in medical settings. In recent years, the development of internalized dispute-resolution mechanisms has only accelerated the translation of ethical questions into legal terms. This reduction of complicated ethical problems to legal matters no doubt makes pragmatic sense. It has, as well, the unfortunate consequence of taking a complicated issue such as who decides the standard of care and translating it into a question of power and authority.

The point here is not that physicians make bad legal philosophers (some do, some do not); rather the point is that a great deal of the world's complexity is washed out when severely compromised neonates are viewed in either technical terms (Can we save this baby?) or legal ones (For what consequences am I liable if I treat or fail to treat, this infant whose life I have the capacity to save?). Entire cultural frames disappear.

Of these, perhaps the most significant is the biographical, familial frame in which parents tend to view their children. If physicians decontextualize infants into organ systems, parents recontextualize them as children in families. Children are beings for whom parents have wishes, dreams, desires, fears, and anxieties. Parents project onto children a role in a family system. Quite literally, parents and physicians talk about children in two different realms of discourse that offer few, if any, points of contact. What is so striking about the cases related above is how inattentive, almost deaf, the physicians are to the parents' concerns (Hunter 1991). Even when the parents are heard, their concerns are seen as human and understandable, but certainly not decisive. Generally, physicians as decision makers need not pay great attention to parental wishes and desires, which are seen as subjective and unreliable (Anspach 1988) or irrelevant (Frader and Bosk 1981).

This point only underscores one more persistent "rough edge" of medical practice: There are simply some fault lines where professional and lay criteria do not meet. Neonatologists measure their craft by their success at salvaging lower and lower birth-weight babies. Follow-up of those babies over the long haul has not been necessary for establishing professional authority. Parents are concerned for a child's healthiness and normality. They measure their fortune or misfortune by how close to the norm their child is. Between these two standards, there is much room for misunderstanding. Each position provides a different warrant for the exercise of decision-making authority. Given how different these warrants are, we might well wonder that there are not more times of open discord between treating physicians and resisting parents.

Public Myth and Private Fears

My task in this chapter was to present two cases where parents sought (and failed) to withdraw treatment over physician objections. These cases illustrate the philosophical and ethical problems in making treatment and nontreatment decisions. What remains is to tie together the description and analysis and to anticipate some likely sources of criticism.

Let us begin with the last task first. The first objection I would raise concerns the narrative framework of the cases discussed. The presentation of the cases does some violence to reality. As the cases unfolded, the events did not emerge quite as neatly as the case presentation here makes it appear. This text is clearly a reconstructed, edited version. The meetings, as they happened, took longer and were less orderly than the narrative discussion implies. Speakers made false starts. Long digressions have been edited out. This editing is quite clearly a potential source of bias. I have turned two meetings in one hospital into stories. Sociologists analyze data; ethnographers do so by interpreting accounts of behavior that they themselves create. Why accept an account from an ethnographic witness?

How do we know they are true stories? The fact that when participants were shown the narrative it accorded with their sense of what happened is hardly comfort. This was how the actors remembered the events. But this is really a weak defense: their memory could be as self-serving as mine. A stronger defense is that narratives are an extraordinarily human way to recall the past. The way parts are arranged into a whole is what creates a tale of social conduct out of an account of mere behavior. The claim for my narrative descriptions is not that they are completely accurate renditions of what happened or the only possible ones. Palmer and Farley, not to mention Bill Smith, all tell very different stories. The claim is more modest: They are a plausible reconstruction, which makes confrontation of certain social dilemmas unavoidable. The goal of the narrative reconstruction is not a phenomenologically perfect snapshot, but an impressionistic sketch—all the better to evoke a response and re-action (Nisbet 1976; Van Maanen 1988).

Even if they are plausible narrative reconstructions, these two cases discuss rare events. Baby Doe situations where a decisive medical intervention will save a life and where the parents are opposed are rare. But underlying conflict between lay persons and professionals is not. Among physicians and patients, the most common cases involve no such disputes over dramatic interven-tion. Those that do are cases that unfold slowly over time, without a clear-cut decisive moment, and with distrust building slowly—a bricolage of missed signals and offhand remarks. These cases are unrepresentative of the complexity of nontreatment issues raised by aggressive treatment of the newborn. One sinks, rather than leaps, into disaster.

To this objection there is a good deal of truth, and the answer to it is not wholly satisfactory. That is to say, Baby Doe cases represent a public myth about the structure of medical care in the hospital con-text. Questions of empirical frequency aside, examining the myth serves to lay bare some of the underlying tensions that beset medi-cal care. The resolution of Baby Doe regulations as a chapter in the bureaucratic regulation of medical practice does not, of course, fully resolve the tensions concerning who is a legitimate decision maker in a nontreatment decision when the patient is incompetent.

Such tensions have entered the public arena in other forms, their presence signaled by case names: Quinlan, Bouvia, Cruzan. That neither of the two cases described here reached such notoriety does not mean that they did not rehearse the same issues. Rather, it indicates that in neither case did the parents want to sacrifice their privacy to make in a public arena their claims of private sovereignty over their child's well being.

5

THE BOUNDARIES OF CARE

The boundaries of care are those of service. As medical professionals, as trained physicians, the genetic counselors defined their obligations as narrowly as they could. For clinic patients, they were experts on diagnoses and recurrence risks. Patients visibly upset by this information were, in the short run, handed over to the clinic coordinator so that they could "ventilate" or "flood out" (Goffman 1961a; Hochschild 1983), those whose emotions needed more "tinkering with" (Goffman 1961a) before a full repair was completed were referred to psychiatry or lay support groups.

Pediatric subspecialists, either residents, fellows, or attending physicians, attempted to funnel "emotions work" to the genetic counselors. Their pride stung, genetic counselors both provided service, as a measurable unit of care (Freidson 1976), and were also able to resist doing the "dirty work" of emotional salvage by invoking their understanding of themselves as "experts" in correctly stating "recurrence risks."

When colleagues attempt to draw counselors into helping with decision making on their clinical problems, they are no more successful than patients are in enlisting such aid for reproductive dilemmas. The genetic counselors' ideology of value-neutrality with respect to outcomes limits the suggestions they make to patients or colleagues for resolving problems.

All of the genetic counselors assume the work they are being asked to do is legitimate. Legitimate requests for service and their management are a "shopfloor indicator" of how a workgroup defines and fulfills its license and mandate—the unique set of tasks and duties that workers claim as their own. A second indicator for examining how license and mandate are defined in everyday situations is the analysis of requests for service that professionals view as illegitimate. Such cases instruct as to the boundaries of the service obligation. This is an interesting question in the case of the genetic counselors, where the service obligation to begin with is framed so narrowly. After all, if one simply states information and avoids directing decision, how can one be called upon improperly for help?

Expertise and Its Boundaries

Legitimate requests for service have two components. First, they acknowledge the specialized knowledge of the genetic counselors. Relative to other physicians who control invasive technologies, the genetic counselors have a limited, if considerably detailed and technical, domain (zone of competence, or sphere of professional authority). At Nightingale Children's Center, genetic counselors inhabit a small niche and are comfortable within it. They are experts at postnatal diagnosis, serving a technical role in the identification of syndromes and chromosomal anomalies. They are also expert at identifying risks prenatally and in recommending strategies to reduce risk and avoid untoward outcomes. The first task they perform at the request of and for other physicians; the second, for patients.

Second, legitimate service requests also respect the value-neutrality with regard to outcomes that genetic counselors stress as the ethical lodestone of their clinical activity. For the genetic counselor, preserving the autonomy of the person—be it colleague or patient—asking the question is important. The genetic counselors define their mission as providing the correct information to colleagues and patients. How that information is used is, of course, consequential but not something that the group intervenes to change through coercive measures. So important is the premium that the genetic counselors place on correct information that they will go to great lengths when they believe that patients have been given information by others that they feel is not technically accurate.

Giordano had invited me to observe a case of his that he thought I, as a sociologist, would find interesting. He described the case as follows. A "young woman of questionable morals with multiple sexual partners and a history of drug use (amphetamines)" had been hospitalized with peritonitis secondary to gonorrhea. During the hospitalization, she was treated with ampicillin and Cleocin. At the time of her treatment, she was pregnant. Both her gynecologist and her internist were strongly opposed to her carrying the baby to term. They told the woman that there was only an 80-percent chance of her having a normal child. They made plans for an abortion and sent the woman a certified letter urging an abortion.

Giordano told me that he felt that these physicians were inappropriately moralizing and that there was no evidence to suggest that Cleocin was such a harmful agent in pregnancy. Giordano said that he told the woman over the phone that she was not at great risk, but he said that he felt that he had to speak to her in person, that he had to offer her personal contact.[1]

After giving me this preamble, Giordano called the woman into the treatment room and began the session: "I called you in to repeat what I told you over the phone."

The Woman: "Yeah."

Giordano: "There are a number of drugs that people take

---

1. The fact that he felt this way underscores how much of a clinician Giordano is, as well as how much a hands-on ethos dominates in definitions of clinical obligations. Giordano had to see his patient to discharge his obligation—there is an irreducible personal element in the doctor-patient relationship satisfied only by mutual physical co-presence. After all, Giordano was not going to reveal anything he had not already told the patient over the phone. Nonetheless, Giordano deemed a meeting necessary, even though this patient needed to travel over ninety minutes just to reach Nightingale.

I am sorry that how this women ever came to ask this question of Giordano in the first place is not something I can reconstruct from my field notes. On her part, however, calling Giordano for an answer to her question was a sensible thing to do. I will not speculate on this point, despite some curiosity now.

I suppose that a reticence to speculate about the empirical details, coupled with delight in speculating about theoretical ones, is what separates the ethnographers from the novelist. If only the fact/theory distinction were an easy one to make, both satisfying ethnographies and novels would be easier to create.

during pregnancy. Now, there are a dozen or so, like thalidomide, that are really dangerous, and we really worry when people take them. Then there are about another half dozen or so that we know are absolutely safe. Most drugs, however, fall somewhere in the middle. They increase your risk but not by that much. Instead of the 2- to 3-percent risk everybody faces, I guess if I had to put a number on it, I'd say that you face a 4- to 5-percent risk."

The Woman: "What about speed? I did some speed. Now I had friends that speeded all during pregnancy. I mean to the very last day. And they delivered perfectly normal babies. I stopped when I found out I was pregnant. So, the way I figure, if they can do that, then a little speed and the one week I spent in the hospital isn't going to do me any harm."

Giordano: "Well, speed is one of those things that we can say has little effect on pregnancy."

The Woman: "I don't know where those people (her internist and obstetrician) get off scaring me the way they did.[2] First, they tell me that I can't have an

2. Giordano agrees. It is the reason he is having this session. At an action level, the two physicians certainly acted clumsily, imperiously, and arrogantly. At the time, I remember being appalled at this attempt to usurp this woman's reproductive autonomy.

Now we are in the midst of a war on drugs, we are more sensitive about the costs of child welfare, we are more aware of the limitations on medical and social resources, and if the woman's use of drugs were intravenous (which is possible, though not likely, given that her drug of choice is amphetamines), we are aware of the health risks of such a pregnancy. So true is this today that had this child been born with defects, this mother would now run some risk of criminal prosecution as a child abuser in some jurisdictions.

Today, we might feel that the two physicians voiced an appropriate concern in an inappropriate manner. They appeared ready to strap her to a table and coerce an abortion against her will. There had to be a better way for them to ask her if she wanted this baby and whether she had thought of its consequences to her and her other two children—a way to ask those questions yet not have it appear as medical terrorism.

Indeed, there must be a way. Unfortunately, it is not prominently on display in the health-care delivery system as it currently operates. But this is not just a problem for the health-care system. I am at a loss here for divining the correct response: one that properly balances risks, responsibilities, and rights. But this confusion is, as I say,

abortion because I might hemorrhage to death all over
the table. Then, they tell me I got to have an abortion
because there is only an 80-percent chance the baby
will be healthy. Hell, I thought, that's great. If it was
serious, like 50/50, maybe then I'd think about having
an abortion. But my philosophy is to live one day at a
time. When the time comes, when the baby's born, if
it's not alright, I'll deal with it then. But I'm not going
to think about it beforehand. The way I figure, this may
be the last baby [she has two other children] I can ever
have because of what was wrong with me in the
hospital, and I really want it. . . ."

Giordano: "As I told you on the phone, I think the other
doctors were just telling you what they would do if
they were in your shoes. But it is your own decision.
You have to make up your own mind. What about the
baby's father? Does he know? Can you talk with him?
Sometimes it helps to have someone as involved as
you are."[3]

Discussion then follows about the woman's social
situation, her relationship to the baby's father, and her
plans to marry another man.[4] The session is then ended.
The woman leaves the room. Giordano turns to me and
says, "Well, she certainly was bizarre. I can see why her
physicians would send her a certified letter, but we have
no business making our patient's decisions for them."

---

recent. Observing the case, I appreciated how far Giordano went to empower and
entitle this woman.

3. I take these questions now to mean that Giordano saw problems with this
woman's decision, while he acknowledges that it was hers to make. The questions
about its consequences, discussed above, fall outside the medical system. Giordano
is trying to lodge them here in the unit of procreation.

4. The woman could not be clearer that the father's feelings are of little concern to
her. She reports that "his jaw just sort of dropped when she told him that there might
be something wrong with the baby". However, since she is going to marry another, it
is "none of his business." Giordano did not ask, and the woman did not elaborate on
how the man she was about to marry felt about the possibility of raising a "damaged"
child; but then, the woman did not speak of him as one she thought would have
much of a role in child rearing.

What is striking about this case is Giordano's definition of the genetic counselor's responsibility, which is to make sure that the woman has factually correct information about reproductive risk, and his failure to explore with her any of the social considerations which might deter her from carrying this pregnancy to term. The service of his colleagues was for Giordano professionally beyond the pale; it provided incorrect information for the purpose of usurping the patient's autonomy. Both the means and the ends of her other physicians were incorrect.

Giordano did not recognize the moralizing element in his response to his colleagues' coercive moralizing for pregnancy termination. In Mark Siegler's (1975) apt description, Giordano's colleagues were "hanging crepe"—they were overstating the riskiness of this pregnancy to the woman. I would characterize Giordano's practice in contrast as "fingerpainting rainbows"— minimizing any risks to this pregnancy. These are the two poles that physicians construct in telling patients the story of their diagnosis. In this case, both ends of the continuum are represented in the two tales told to a single patient. In each case the story the physicians constructed told the patient what to do (although Giordano did so obliquely and indirectly). In neither case did the physicians explore what the patient wanted to do or why. Both responses moralize; all that differs is where the moralizing leads. Neither response invites a dialogue. Neither Giordano nor his colleagues are to be blamed for declining the opportunity for colloquy. Since talk is both cheap and difficult to bill for, involvement here multiplies the opportunity for trouble without any hope of reward. The genetic counselors recognize that their "risk figures" provide many couples with permission to continue a pregnancy, but the manner in which they do this—"just providing accurate information"— they consider absent of any moralizing component. Moreover, they resist patients' attempts to get them to interpret the numbers, for this is the "essence" of moralizing, of telling patients what to do.

As they go about their work, a constant refrain of the counselors is that the standard for good work is not the patient's decision but the information they provide to the patient for making that decision. When pressed by patients for recommendations, the genetic counselors, as noted above, refuse to give them.

Samuels is counseling the Bagleys, a couple who have
come in for counseling because Mrs. Bagley's brother has
just had a child die from anencephaly. It is the end of the
counseling session. Samuels has given the couple their
risk figures and explained about prenatal diagnosis. As
Samuels is ready to close the session, he asks if there are
any further questions.

Mr. Bagley says, "Just one, what are your own personal
recommendations for us?"

Samuels answers, "It's not our policy at the center to
give you recommendations. It's really a matter of what
you can live with and what you can't live with. Say you
have a baby without the test, and the baby has a problem;
then you may have wanted the test. Say you have a baby
with the test, and the baby turns out to be okay; then you
may think testing is silly. Or say you have the test and lose
the pregnancy; you may blame that on the test. It is really
just a matter of what course of action you are most
comfortable with. Some people that are in your shoes just
have the blood test, some decide to do nothing, and some
decide to have amniocentesis."

Mr. Bagley asks, "Are these people with our risk?"

Samuels says, "Yes;[5] it is not clear what you should do.
There is a gray area. No, it's not so much a gray area as a
personal thing."

To this, Mr. Bagley responds, "I just don't want to make
a big mistake."

Samuels reassures him, "You can't make a mistake for

5. Samuels's yes here is quite extraordinary in that it cuts against the grain of standard practice. More commonly, the genetic counselors challenge the premise of the
Bagleys' question. They deny that there as another couple like the Bagleys in their
values, their goals, their upbringing. Every couple is different, so no two couples
ever have to make the same decision.

The fact that Samuels "broke frame" (Goffman 1974) to the extent that he did
invites speculation as to what it was about the Bagleys that evoked a response in
Samuels. Beyond the specific question is a more general, weighty one for students of
service organizations: In a bureaucratic organization, what makes some cases special and worthy of extra consideration? For an intriguing discussion of special cases
in the juvenile justice system see Jacobs (1990).

you. If you do what you are comfortable with, then it is
the right decision."

Samuels' reassurance here is intriguing, in light of the conversational time he spent outlining all the ways a decision can later be
seen as mistake, depending on its consequences. But this emphasis
on private, personal values serves to limit both his involvement in
and responsibility for outcomes. It limits the domain of the genetic
counselors' task to the quality of the technical information they provide. Moreover, it would appear that if the Bagleys can't make a mistake so long as they make a decision that is "right for them," then
neither can Samuels, so long as the recurrence risk he provided
was factually correct.

The fact that genetic counselors absent themselves from patient
decision making helps explain some peculiar findings in the literature on how patients use the information they receive in genetic counseling. Hoffmaster (1990) has recently reinterpreted
Lippman-Hand and Fraser's (1979) study of parental decision making after genetic counseling.

> Their [Lippman-Hand and Fraser's] research was, in other
> words, designed to assess the adequacy of genetic coun-
> seling in terms of an influential philosophical method of
> moral decision making [rational utilitarianism]. What they
> discovered, to their surprise, is that patients uniformly
> ignore the probabilities of alternative outcomes. They
> reduce the problems to two results—either we will have
> a defective child or we will not have a defective child.
> They then construct scenarios of what it would be like to
> live with a defective child, and if they think they could
> cope with the worst of these scenarios, they run the risk
> of conceiving a child who might be handicapped.

Lippman-Hand and Fraser's research documents how, at one
level, genetic counseling fails to work—those precise risk figures
gathered at such great price hardly play a role in patient decision
making. On another level, however, the research documents how
successful genetic counselors have been in achieving the goal of
preserving the patient as the responsible decision maker.

The fact that the onus of decision making falls to patients is something that the genetic counselors remind themselves of whenever there is uncertainty, doubt, or conflict in the group about what a couple should do.

At the postclinic conference, Giordano is discussing his session with the Stones. Mrs. Stone is pregnant, and her amniocentesis had an equivocal result. She is suspected of having a supranumerary marker.

Giordano reported that the session was "very strange." The husband, who is "very methodical, an accountant, was listing the pros and cons for having an abortion." But the couple was still very uncertain about what to do. Giordano said that he could have made their problem easier, made the problem more resolvable, by being more definitive. What he did do was impose a Monday deadline for a decision (it is now Friday), and he said he gave them a 10-percent risk for having a child with some appreciable defect, because they asked for and needed a number in order to make a decision.

Samuels, on hearing this, objected to the way Giordano had managed the couple. "I don't know where you got that number from. It's clear that they have an increased risk, but it's impossible to place a precise number on it. We have a clinical finding that's associated with an unknown anomaly. We know that their risk is higher [then normal] but we have no reason to say that it's 10 percent. I think in this kind of counseling situation, you have to give the couple more direction."

To Samuels's objection, Bill Smith had objections of his own, which he expressed in a cascade of questions, "What do you mean more direction? Do you mean we should make their minds up for them? Should we tell them what to do? What direction would you counsel them in?"

Samuels knew exactly what direction he would take in counseling. He described the pregnancy as "unacceptable" and then continued: "The woman is thirty-four, she had the procedure done for high anxiety, and nothing that has been done so far would reduce the level of anxiety. In fact, given the marker, this is the kind of situation where you can't even tell immediately after birth whether or not the child will be born with some damage."

Giordano objected to Samuels's characterization of the case as requiring more "direction." He said he viewed the situation the "same as any woman who came in with an undiagnosable condition that had a risk attached to it, say cystic fibrosis."[6]

Samuels argued with the appropriateness of this analogy: "I just don't think it's analogous. You have a test result. And when you look at the whole picture, the thirty-four-year-old woman, the high anxiety—you see she needs more direction. You have a resolvable situation; you can remove her anxiety by performing the abortion. And if you told her she could get pregnant again, they wouldn't be in the place they are now."

Giordano responds with a correct statement of clinic policy, "But we don't accept this burden in other situations; we don't tell our patients what to do then. Why should I accept the onus of telling them to abort. Look, if this were a case of trisomy 16, I'd have no trouble letting them off the hook, but I can't do that. The finding here is associated with severe defects occasionally, but I can't say for certain that the child is defective. I don't know why I should be directive in this case when I wouldn't be in other cases."

Samuels's objection to Giordano's lack of direction is interesting on a number of counts. First, recall Samuels's own equivocation

---

6. Another advance since these field materials were gathered: Cystic fibrosis is no longer undiagnosable. This development, like the one with Huntington's, has amplified uncertainties at another level.

when the Bagleys asked for his personal recommendation. In that session he brushed off the patient's request for direction by a blanket statement that honoring such requests violated the policy of the Center. Next, of all the members of the genetics team, it was Giordano, whose high-risk obstetric practice required exacting clinical decisions, who was most comfortable giving patients orders. As Bill Smith once put it, "Only Giordano will walk into a room and say, 'I'm the doctor and this is what you should do.'"

Samuels's call for direction carried little weight. No one else at the conference seconded it. It was noteworthy as well for its rareness. It could have been said about any session that couples could or should have been given more direction. Yet this rarely occurred. This was one of the few public disagreements (to which I was privy) over a couple being given too little direction. In fact, no one in the group believed that direction was what genetic counselors were supposed to supply. As they saw it, their charge was to provide accurate information, and this was constantly reiterated whenever the occasion presented itself.

> At the postclinic conference, Berger reported on seeing the parents of a child who had just been born with an open myelomeningocele. The parents had decided to place the child in a residential home and had decided not to repair the neural-tube defect. Berger first reported that he did "standard" myelo counseling.
>
> He then reported some more on the parents. He said the mother is a gardener who's around insecticides a lot; she had some questions about whether any of these agents would have contributed to the birth defect. The father, Berger reported, was difficult to read.
>
> The parents, continued Berger, were comfortable with the decision not to treat, and did not want to rethink it. They were "leery" of today's session because somewhere along the line "they had been exposed to someone who had challenged the decision, perhaps a sister-in-law."
>
> The sister-in-law had brought in parents of children who had decided to make the repair. From them, the

parents had received the "classic" build-up of the child
who may do alright in the end. Nonetheless, the parents
did not change their minds and did not want to discuss
their decision further.

Berger said that it was not the task of the Unit to have
them do so. "Our job here is not to convince parents to
do one thing or the other. We provide information. We
make sure that they are comfortable with what it is that
they are going to do."

Berger's explicit announcement of the group's mission is particularly noteworthy because he is both its most senior member and its
formal leader. Also, it presents a paradox: How, if the parents did
not want to discuss their decision, could Berger evaluate if they
were comfortable with it? In fact, does not the parents' insistence
on keeping the lid to this particular Pandora's Box closed speak to
a certain level of discomfort? There is an interactional contradiction that inheres in the practice of genetic counseling. A commitment to nondirection requires a certain reticence to explore
issues that patients keep closed. Yet a commitment to decisions
that "patients are comfortable with" requires a certain amount of
unpleasant prying if only to assure that the comfort presented is
genuine.

The genetic counselors evaluated their performance in terms of
the story that they told parents. They judged the stories (Did they
reflect the current state of genetic knowledge?), but not the story-
telling. Whether the stories they fashioned acted as effective moral
parables, as guides to patient action, remained a mystery. The genetic counselors made no efforts to see if parents understood those
stories. They did not ask parents to repeat their understandings;
they did not schedule follow-ups after those sessions where they
felt that parents had incorrectly interpreted what they were told.
The emphasis on "the telling" and not "the hearing" is itself an example of a more general tendency of professionals to evaluate their
work in terms of process not outcomes. In fact, any attempts to link
outcomes and efficacy were explicitly disavowed.

Giordano is presenting a case at the preclinic conference.
The Bensons (like the Stones, who were discussed
above) have an equivocal finding on amniocentesis; it is
another chromosomal mosaicism. He says, "Look, we've
been in this situation before with Mrs. Whatsit, who had
the funny third chromosome. We downplayed it, and
everything worked out happily; things worked out in that
situation."

At this point, Bill Smith says, "You've got to watch that."

Giordano is puzzled, "Watch what?"

Bill said, "That 'happily'—what if the Whatsits aborted,
and the fetus had been normal? Well, it still would have
been 'happily' because it was a situation they could live
with." Bill then said that Giordano should avoid saying
'happily' for pregnancies that are carried to term, that
that's not necessarily anymore of a happy conclusion than
an abortion, that the important thing is to see that the
families got good counseling, not whether or not their
pregnancies were carried to term.

Giordano defended himself by saying that he said
'happily' because it worked out that way. He then added,
"I'm the least squeamish person in the room about
aborting Mrs. Benson, and if, at the same time, she elects
to keep her pregnancy, then I'm not about to go jumping
off the West End Bridge."

Bill Smith responded, "We're beyond jumping off
bridges now."

As a group, genetic counselors are beyond jumping off bridges, in
this case, because they have crossed one attitudinally. Decision
making in reproductive matters is a private, not a medical matter.
This is why Samuels's suggestion of aggressively pursuing abortion
in the "marker" case of Giordano is so roundly rejected. Here, ironically, contact with professionals who are strangers in the context of
a formal organization, the pediatric hospital, functions to preserve
privacy. But this is not an inevitable outcome; a different work ideology and set of shopfloor practices might generate a very different
result.

Beyond the Bounds of Expertise

Technical, scientific information was always provided without any reticence, provided the person asking the question was a person who could legitimately ask the question. This was so even if the information itself was of little relevance, even if it was presented so that it could be ignored.

> The Conroys have come in for counseling. Mrs. Conroy is pregnant. They have one healthy child, and recently Mrs. Conroy gave birth to a child who died at six and one-half months. The pattern of malformation had created a suspicion of trisomy 13.
>
> The genetic counselors have worked the child up. A holoprozencephalyl recessive genetic error had not caused the anencephaly; there was no evidence of any chromosomal problem. The parents, who have been counseled before, want to hear about the recurrence risk for the disease.
>
> Giordano begins the session: "Well, I hear you have good news for us."
> *Mrs. Conroy:* "Yes, I'm pregnant."[7]
> *Giordano:* "How do you feel about that?"
> *Mrs. Conroy:* "Well, I'm glad and very anxious. It was unplanned. I had an IUD, and we weren't planning to have a child, and now I guess I'm anxious."
>
> Giordano said that it was understandable for Mrs. Conroy to be anxious and asks why they had come in today.
>
> Mr. Conroy answers, "Well, we'd like to run over what we talked about before. I guess because of the situation, we weren't really listening. Now, we'd like to get it all straight in our heads."
>
> Giordano smiles and says, "Sure, Stacey had a very rare disease. It has multiple causes. One of those may be chromosomal damage, but we did tests and ruled that out. Various drugs in animals have been shown to cause

---

7. Note Giordano's behavior as an obstetrician: pregnancy is framed as good news.

this disorder, but we don't think that was the case with Stacey. Third, sometimes we don't know what causes it in most cases, nor do we know its incidence. . . . Whatever, it is presumably a very rare gene, and the chances of it being genetic with you are very small. Overall, I would say that your chances are between 0 and 25 percent."

Giordano then takes a piece of paper from the chart and draws two boxes connected by a line. In the box on the left margin, he places a zero. In the one on the right, a twenty-five. He explains that most cases of the disease fall in the zero box. He estimates the Conroys' overall risk at 4 percent, but cautions them, "There is no guarantee that you will have a perfect child. There is never any guarantee that you will have a perfect child."

Mr. Conroy asks, "Is there any way to predetermine if the child has this condition."

Giordano tells them there is not and once again runs through the conditional probabilities and asks how the couple are feeling about the pregnancy. They mention their anxiety again. Giordano reassures them.

The session seems to be winding down. Mrs. Conroy appears ready to leave. She says, "We know we've heard all this before. We just needed to hear it again. We wanted to hear it again.

Giordano says, "You shouldn't feel embarrassed about that." He then goes on: "Now, there is no way to test for the gene or the defect. But there is something you should know about. I think it is impractical, but I have to tell you that it exists. There is this test—they are doing it at Three-Hundred-Miles-North-of-Here Medical Center—there is this test where you take an instrument the size of this (he points to a thermometer), and you insert it with a local anesthetic into the uterus and try to look at the parts of the fetus you are interested in seeing. It's very, very experimental. It's been done only about, perhaps, thirty times. And I think there is a great chance of risk to the pregnancy. The chances of loss or injury are high. Now, the kind of defect we are talking about here potentially can be seen. If we knew that you had a 25 percent recurrence risk, we would consider it. But I think your risk of having a child with Stacey's problems are much less than the risks of the procedure. And if I were you, I don't think you would want to consider it. Now it is true that some people use testing as a means of reassurance, but even then the numbers are unchanged. With this test there is an awful lot that we don't know—such as what are the effects of shining a bright light into the uterus, which is, after all, supposed to be a dark place. If you want, I'll get information. But this is nothing that I want to push."

Mr. Conroy says that they are uninterested in pursuing this test [fetoscopy], and Mrs. Conroy asks Giordano to send a summary of the session to her obstetrician.

Giordano's discussion of fetoscopy as a highly experimental procedure which he does not recommend is puzzling. First, why does he mention it, if it is so highly experimental and he is so negative? Second, does not his way of discussing direct the parents not to exercise this option; does it not violate the genetic counselor's goal of nondirective sessions? For Giordano, not to mention the test would have been to fail to be complete. It would have violated the unit's ethos by not mentioning the cutting edge of prenatal diagnosis. The Conroys needed to "hear" about the test, but they also needed to hear that it was not a reasonable option.

But it is not only the latest technical information that the genetic counselors as clinicians feel obligated to tell those who use their services; it is their options as well. After all, in the second Baby Doe case discussed in the previous chapter, it was the neonatologist's decision to raise, out of a sense of obligation to completeness, the option (which was "not really an option") of nontreatment to Mr. Flannery that led to that father's seventy-two hour resistance to consent. During the backstage discussion of this case, Bill Smith and the neonatologists spent a great deal of time defending that disclosure as necessary. At the same time, Palmer and the surgeons used an equal and competing block of time in criticizing it. Stating options does not always amount to the neutral provision of advice. Some options have the force of a directive (i.e., your money or your life). Once counselors act to frame options for their clients, a certain contradictoriness creeps in between occupational principles of neutrality and occupational practices.

Although the counselors also feel obligated to include all reproductive options in counseling sessions, so that parents will hear a complete story, it was clear that some of these options were not to be discussed today; that they were part of another professional group's turf. These included artificial insemination by a donor as a way to avoid autosomal recessive disorders. The genetic counselors told parents it was something that "they might want to think about." If they were interested, the parents should contact the genetic counselors, who would then refer them to the proper resources. To cover all bases, the genetic counselors also felt obliged to raise adoption as a child-rearing option. But the difficulties with adoption introduced a note of extreme caution into the discussion. The possibility of choosing to remain childless was mooted by the professional task: counseling about reproductive risks.

The genetic counselors also felt obligated to tell parents of children affected by genetic anomalies that they might want or have to think about residential placement of "hard-to-manage" disabled children. Again this was mentioned by the genetic counselors in a way that signaled it was not part of today's agenda. Finally, a third category of topics that counselors felt obligated to raise to parents who expressed difficulty in coping with a situation was the availability of support services. This included a ritualistic injunction that "talking helps." The category of people with whom "talking" might be particularly helpful included family, "people who have gone through something similar" (especially those connected with organized support groups), clergy, and mental health professionals. Professionals were the last and least-mentioned category of those with whom it might be useful to talk. In part, this reflected the genetic counselors' protection of patient sensitivities. Aware of the persistent public prejudice against and stigma attached to mental health treatment, the counselors do not want to offend parents.

Also aware of health insurance difficulties associated with benefits for mental health services, the genetic counselors do not want to extend false hope for help. Further, their own difficulty (discussed in chapter 3) at triaging the patients they see who display the most florid signs of emotional disturbance makes the genetic counselors skeptical about the efficacy of mental health services for milder forms of upset.

Finally, it is interesting to note that the genetic counselors always omitted themselves from the list of people with whom talk is helpful. Experts at recurrence risks, the genetic counselors even so included the obligation to tell a complete story in their definition of their clinical role. There are, nonetheless, times when the counselors fail to do so. Sometimes this occurs because they are not certain how much right the person asking the question has to raise it.

> I arrive at clinic early and ask the clinic coordinator, Nancy Thomas, what's on tap. She says, "Not much; Bill's meeting with a lawyer at 1:00, but you wouldn't be interested in that. Al's got a cystic family at 2:00, and Joe's got a couple of pre-amnios." Nancy is wrong about my interest in the lawyer. This is the case I ask to observe.
>
> Bill asks the lawyer, who represents a mother whose child Bill diagnosed as having trisomy 21, "How can we help you?"
>
> The lawyer begins, "So you won't be disturbed or defensive about me being here, let me tell you where we stand with this case. This is, for our firm, a case of medical malpractice. The litigation involves the claim that the obstetrician did not live up to the standards of practice in the community and that he should have advised Mrs. McKenna, who was forty-one in 1974, at the time of her pregnancy of her increased risks for the possibility of a child with mental retardation, of the possibility of prenatal diagnosis, of the fact that in theory a child with Down's syndrome was discoverable, and of the option of terminating the pregnancy. We are going, in this case, to avoid the question of what she would have done. It is not

germane to argue about whether or not she would have terminated the pregnancy.[8] We have retained experts who will say what should have been done in this case."

Bill asks, "Can I know what they said?"

The lawyer passes him the letters of four expert witnesses, three from New York, one from the medical center of which Nightingale is a part.

Bill reads the letters and points out that the registry data establishing the safety and efficacy of amniocentesis was not published until 1976.

The lawyer responds, "You know, so much of the law has to do with informed consent, and we are really trying to get away from the community standard area and try the case on the grounds of informed consent. Mrs. McKenna tells us that she asked the obstetrician if her age represented any increased risk to the baby in pregnancy, and she says he said, 'No, you'll drop it like a twenty-three-year-old,' and that he didn't say anything to her about the increased risk of mental retardation. Now, the doctor's lawyer, hearing of Mrs. McKenna's statements, said that what we have here is a question of credibility. They haven't raised the question of whether or not amniocentesis was being done in the community. They say they were already doing amniocentesis then. They claim that they told her about amniocentesis, and she knew about the risk and was adequately informed by them."

Bill says, "You could prove that."

The lawyer mentions that they've subpoenaed the records and that they show that all amniocenteses were done later than this, but their [the doctor's] lawyers still claim that we recommended amniocentesis to her and

---

8. My reading of Canterbury v. Spence, 474 F.2d 772 (1976), is that the lawyer is wrong here. It is very much germane in a malpractice action what the plaintiff would have done had he or she known. When this classic informed-consent case was retired, the jury found for the defendant, Dr. Spence, chiefly, one suspects, because the nondisclosure was not material to Mr. Canterbury. This finding was upheld on appeal (Epstein, Gregory, and Kolven 1984, 188).

talked to her. He then adds, "The real reason I came here
today, Doctor, was to see if you could, from your notes,
your reaction [to your] notes rather than the notes
themselves, tell me anything about Faith McKenna that
struck you as interesting about your first contacts."

Bill looks over his notes and tells the lawyer, "It says
here that the pediatrician referred the baby saying that its
eyes were funny, that it had a thick neck, lots of mucous,
and its tongue was out. It appears that we saw them on
9/28, and my ward notes note that my impressions are
consistent with Down's syndrome, that we drew blood,
and that we discussed amnio, and that's it."

The lawyer continues: "I guess you see a lot of people,
Dr. Smith, but would you remember if she indicated to you
that she had heard about it [amniocentesis]? My hope in
coming here today is that you would have some
recollection of Mrs. McKenna, something would jog your
memory, and you would be able to tell me when I asked,
she said, 'Oh, my God, why didn't they tell me that!' or
even 'I know about that—my obstetrician told me about
the test, and I decided not to do it.' But something that
one way or another could help with credibility.[9] The
McKennas are clients, no they are more than clients, they
have become friends, and I think Faith makes a creditable
witness, but I was hoping to find something that would
nail it down one way or the other."

Bill says, "Let me tell you where I'm at. I don't want to
make up a story for you. I don't want to fabricate
something. I have a great deal of difficulty telling a family
they have a child with Down's syndrome and telling them
what it means. That means I have a great deal of trouble
in terms of telling the right way, in a way that stays and
remains with them. Now, in a case like this, where the
mother is forty-one, when I don't know if the woman
knew about amniocentesis and how she would react if it

9. For a discussion of the lawyer's interview strategy and a comparison of it with
the physician's, see Scheff's interesting article (1968).

was denied her, I'm walking on eggshells. The only thing
I can tell you is that I did a physical exam the same day I
did a blood test, and that means they were "anxious."

The lawyer asks, "Then there is nothing about the
McKennas that you remember one way or the other?"

Bill answers, "No, as I said, I was walking on eggshells,
and when I'm walking on those eggshells and I
have to bring up the probability of the next child to a
woman that's forty-one years old, I've worked out a way of
dealing with it, what I call a *routine,* and I stick with that
routine, which emphasizes three points: first, that the test
is available; two, that it can be done here; and three, that
there is an increased risk of having another child with
Down's syndrome with maternal age. I make sure to
emphasize that risk is statistical, and we don't know
whose fault it is, that is, where it occurs. I try to make sure
that I don't put the blame on either parent. Now in the
midst of that I end up not remembering the actual
responses of the parents. I'm often too anxious to pay any
attention to it."

The lawyer leaves the question of consent and asks Bill
about the question of damages—what special services
the child would require.

Bill says, "I'm comfortable saying that the child will
need special school. Understand, I'm not volunteering.
But I think that the chart indicates that the child has a
heart defect. If you want to know about any special
problems the child has, you should go to the cardiologist
and ask him point blank. Now maybe you will bring about
a whole Pandora's Box, because he may not have told the
parents. They also may not be ready to hear. There's a
good chance that the cardiologist hasn't told the family
anything yet. They tend to avoid that and play things in a
day-to-day fashion." Bill then asks the lawyer to send a
photograph of the McKennas "to see if it jogs his
memory."

The lawyer promises to do so and leaves. When he
does, Bill rounds on me. He tells me that he thinks he

remembers that the mother was surprised, but that he
would be uncomfortable saying so in court because
he doesn't know for sure, and he has no record of
it. He's quite upset that the lawyer has come to ask
him. He complains that it puts him in a very
uncomfortable position. Then he complains about the
process of being a witness and the considerable loss of
time it entails.

At the postclinic conference, after Bill discusses the
session, Giordano comments that now whenever a
woman comes in for amniocentesis counseling, he sends
a letter to the referring obstetrician to protect against just
this kind of suit.

I have related this case in great detail for a number of reasons.
First, there are Bill Smith's statements about both what he hopes to
accomplish when counseling parents about Down's syndrome and
how he feels about it. Second, there is the opportunity to observe
interprofessional relations in a sensitive and difficult area, first-
hand. Third, there is the notable difference in candor between what
Bill is willing to tell the lawyer and what he is willing to tell me.
There are a number of reasons why he is not more forthcoming,
not the least of which is his awareness of what complete candor
would entail for him later. Even so, had the lawyer asked him to
testify or "be a witness" on a technical matter, Bill might have
agreed to do so. Although it is a bother, Bill is willing to act as a
witness in his area of expertise. Here, Bill did not feel the same obligation he did to a patient to tell a "complete story." The complete
story that the lawyer was after went beyond Bill's professionally
trained capacities. Noting reactions and gauging emotional responses are outside of the genetic counselors' frame of reference.
However much they serve as societal witnesses, there are quite
clearly limits to this role for the genetic counselors. Finally, there is
the way Bill's resentment at the indignities of being a witness rever-
berated with my discovery of my role as ethnographic witness and
with my own growing sense of anger and impatience at the role's
limitations.

Bill Smith's problems with the lawyer reappear in other guises as the counselors go about their routine work. One noteworthy instance occurs when, in the counselor's eyes, the person asking the question is not necessarily entitled to an answer. On numerous occasions, the parents of retarded children asked the genetic counselors to meet with their children to help dissuade them from bearing children. The genetic counselors felt such work to be outside the domain of their expertise. First, they were not, as they often reminded themselves, in the business of deciding who should and who should not have children. Second, the counseling enterprise broke down when the consumers of the probabilistic information about pregnancy risks could not be counted on to be instrumental and rational problem solvers. Finally, the counselors found it uncomfortable to talk to the retarded about having a retarded child. They did so, nonetheless, with normal parents present. Genetic counseling for the "mutually differently abled" poses a problem for genetic counselors. It is often unclear if what the couple desires is offspring who are "the same" as them or offspring who are different.[10]

Occasionally parents who were opposed to their children's selection of mates sent their children to genetic counselors. The parents' expectation was that in the face of rational scientific arguments, their children could overcome their sentimental attachments. If the couple showed up, the counselors generally gave a complete story. In this vein, an engaged couple was counseled about the inheritance of schizophrenia.[11] However, on those rare occasions when parents showed up with a grown child and asked about the genetic risks of that child's intended, then the genetic counselors suspended the rule of candor.

> I was observing one of Samuels's cases. A mother and
> father had brought in their daughter for counseling.
> Samuels asked to see the daughter alone first.

10. I am grateful to Anne Steinberg for that observation, gleaned from her experience in the deaf community.

11. Here the counseling disturbed me—a sociologist with an interest in deviance and labeling theory—since it elided so many of the difficulties in defining schizophrenia and its etiology. The couple, nonetheless, was reassured by (even if during the interview confused about) the empiric risk figures they were given.

He asked her, "What do you know, and what do you want to know?"

The daughter, who was crying, explained that her boyfriend's father had a disease, where he couldn't walk, couldn't work, and her parents were worried that if she married the boyfriend, her whole life was going to be caring for him. She added that the father's disease was genetic.

Samuels asked, "Who told you it was a genetics problem?"

The daughter explained that her parents had contacted the boyfriend's father and gotten permission to get his medical records. They had discussed these with their family physician and with a relative who was also a physician. From the records, they found out that the boy's father had Friederich's ataxia. The daughter explained that her parents had done this behind her back and that her physician cousin had said they should break up. She said this was confusing to her, because the boy's own doctor had said that he had nothing to worry about. She said the boyfriend never talked about the problem and didn't seem too worried about it.

Samuels responded, "Well, it's very hard to do anything without your boyfriend here. We now have a new name for the father's problem. It is Roussy-Levy's syndrome. In some ways that's just as bad. It is a dominant genetic disorder and that means that there is a 50-percent chance your boyfriend has it. If he has it, there is a 50-percent chance of passing it on to any children." Samuels then goes on to explain variable degrees of expression: how the father could be severely affected, but the son only mildly affected. Whatever was the case, they wouldn't know until the boyfriend was evaluated by a neurologist.

The daughter continued to cry, and asked, "Then nothing can be done without telling him?" Samuels nodded, yes. The daughter became more distraught and began to talk, "What if his mother doesn't want him to know? Now my parents saw his father, and he never sees him. Suppose his mother made his physician promise never to tell him anything about the disease, and we've now gone behind his back?"

Samuels weathered the daughter's affect storm and said, "If your feelings for him are deep and his for you likewise, and if you explain your concerns, then he should be only too willing to see a neurologist. It doesn't make sense to think that his mother should forbid him to know; that's not something that a mother can do. I'm going to call your parents in now, and we can all talk together; but I want to remind you that this is your decision, not theirs."

Samuels fetched the parents and asked them to tell him "their major concerns."

The mother began, "Our concern is hereditary. When her boyfriend told us his father had Friederich's ataxia, we called a relative and our doctor. They said it was a hereditary problem and Jill should break it off."

Samuels responded, "Heredity seems to have a bad name in your family. It's not a question of heredity— intelligence is inherited; there are a lot of things that are inherited, good things as well as bad things. It's a question of consequences—how bad they are and whether you can manage them."

Samuels then talked to the parents, repeating what he had said to the daughter, that nothing definitive could be said unless the boyfriend was present, that diseases have different forms of expression, and that they needed to respect their daughter's judgment.

The session ended with the parents promising to invite Samuels to the wedding "If everything worked out."

Samuels's conduct of this session is interesting for a number of reasons. First, the medical records that he has indicated that the boyfriend already has the disease. Both the age of onset and the father's condition do not bode well for the boyfriend's future. Hence his discussion of variable expression held out a false hope to the girlfriend. Enough hope, Samuels hoped, would propel her to the next stage: a visit with a neurologist. Nonetheless, Samuels does not feel he can reveal this either without confirming the record by examining the boy or without the boy's permission. He is not about to violate patient confidentiality because a couple of parents object to the suitability of their seventeen-year-old daughter's boyfriend. While Samuels tells a complete story about Roussy-Levy in the abstract, he does not do so for this concrete situation. For him, it would be a serious breach of medical ethics to do so. Thus, genetic counselors are committed to telling a complete story, but only to those entitled to hear it. This includes only those with reproductive or treatment decisions premised on this information. It does not extend to interested third parties like lawyers or unhappy, but very involved, parents.

The rule of complete candor is also suspended on one other occasion: namely, when an option is open to couples, but that option is not socially acceptable. There are things we can imagine but do not do. There is no compelling need to talk with couples about speculative possibilities not available through conventional social arrangements.

> We are in postclinic conference. Bill Smith has just
> described his session with a couple with Huntington's
> chorea. The wife's mother is the affected person;
> consequently, the wife has a 50-percent chance of
> inheriting the disease, and if she does so, a 50-percent
> chance of passing it on.
>
> Someone in the group asks why these couples
> consider pregnancy at all—the rational strategy being, in
> the questioner's eyes, simply to forbear from having
> children.
>
> Berger delivers a little homily about childbearing
> being a form of denial and that refusing to have children
> is a little too frank an acknowledgment that you might get
> the disease.
>
> When Berger finishes, Samuels asks an interesting
> question: "With the shortage of babies for adoption, how
> come we never consider the idea of a surrogate uterus?"

Samuels then produced an article from that day's paper about a woman in California who was acting as a surrogate mother. [This discussion is being held six years before Mary Beth Whitehead's celebrated case.]

At first, Samuels's suggestion is met by much anxious laughter from all the members of the group. Then, one by one, each member of the group suggested that in many ways this seemed to be a "reasonable alternative."

Members of the group were hard-pressed to make a distinction between artificial insemination of the wife where recessive disease is present, or where the husband is infertile.

Berger felt that there was a great difference between having a mother artificially inseminated and having another woman carry the child around for nine months. Nonetheless, the group was struck by the fact that here was a rational solution to many of the problems they faced that was nowhere offered to couples. They all agreed that the only thing preventing it was an "ingrained male-chauvinist attitude about the sacredness of pregnancy."

Despite feelings that this might in many cases be a reasonable alternative, they decided that the center was not going to mention it as an alternative, because society was not ready to deal with it, and because the logistical problems involved were bound to be considerable. They felt their work was difficult enough without adding this new wrinkle to it.

The genetic counselors' discussion in some ways represented the best politically correct thinking of the time: Principles of androgyny were extended to reproduction. In principle, formal equality is upheld; who contributes what in the reproductive process is irrelevant. If men can be surrogates, so can women. Our conventional wisdom is now more gendered; we recognize the special bonding of mother and progeny. In fact, Fletcher and Evans (1983) have shown that modern prenatal diagnosis deepens the attachment of mother and fetus. A good surrogacy contract would require frequent monitoring, increasing the attachment of the surrogate to the child she bears for another couple. The judgment of the genetic counselors that society was not ready to deal with surrogate mothers has certainly been vindicated by cases like the Whitehead one, which equated the practice of surrogacy with baby-selling. The New Jersey Supreme Court ruled that surrogacy was a commercial transaction that involved too many regulatory problems to be worth the social benefits. The court still makes room for forms of loving surrogacy, signaling its recognition of the difference between public, economic transactions and private, affective ones.

This was not the only technological possibility that the genetic counselors failed to mention to prospective parents. A second area of structured silence concerned sex selection of fetuses following amniocentesis. On this matter the center, unlike some others, which explicitly forbade sex selection, did not have a formal policy. On two occasions parents consulted the center about sex selection. Rather than refusing to consider either of these two cases, the genetic counselors decided to deal with them on an ad hoc basis, acknowledging that there were situations other than X-linked disorders in which they could imagine fetal sex as being a legitimate reason for pregnancy termination. In both cases, amniocentesis was performed, and both pregnancies were carried to term. In both cases, the couples stated that they would not terminate a pregnancy for sex selection; but of course the genetic counselors lacked a compliance mechanism. Had the women wished to abort, the genetic counselors were prepared to take a "let's talk, then decide" stance.

Reproduction as a Private Arena

What is interesting about each of these last two examples is that they involve areas of significant public-policy controversy. Surrogate motherhood and the sex selection of fetuses are each viewed as dangers posed by the new reproductive technologies. As Kass (1972) has pointed out, this sort of tinkering with the old, reproductive methods threatens to alter at a basic level our conception of parenthood, the family, and individual identity. The genetic counselors were well aware of these threats. They were aware as well of the controversies that surrounded the reproductive rights of the retarded, second-trimester abortions, and the excessive reliance on genetic background for decision making about marriage.

Nonetheless, the counselors adopted as a strategy for managing all these difficult issues one which chose to ignore the collective implications of genetic practice. Instead, they focused on their interactions with patients as a private transaction. Patients were given complete stories when they were entitled to them and were encouraged to make up their own minds. Others who sought out the genetic counselors' advice, but who were not seen as doing so legitimately, were not met with stony silence, but they were not given full stories either.

The larger societal debate about abortion was never allowed to intrude on the clinic in any direct way, yet its indirect effects were many. Most notably, the restrictions on public funding of abortions limited the clinic population to those with private insurance. This raises for me great questions about equity. Extensive, expensive, high-technology care is available to the pregnant middle-class woman, while the most rudimentary care is often not provided to the least-privileged members of the society. What is a fundamental right for those with private health insurance is denied to those whose health care is contingent on public funds. Observing the genetic counselors at Nightingale is to watch closely one tier only of a two-tiered health-care system. The group would pass through waiting areas crowded with one tier's clients—the black, urban poor—on its way to provide service to the other tier, a collection of employed and insured white men and women.

Next, there was great squeamishness about the possibility of false positives from amniocentesis, and this was so despite the potential legal costs of being wrong. Recall in this context the debate between Samuels and his colleagues over the advisability of recommending abortion to the woman with a supranumerary marker. Recall as well the emphasis on amniocentesis as a device for reassurance. Finally, the insistence on patient autonomy and private decision making was itself observed to operate in an asymmetric fashion. The genetic counselors felt free to give encouragement about maintaining pregnancies, but retreated behind neutrality when the issue was ending them.

The autonomy that genetic counselors accord their patients means that the reasons that couples give for their decisions are not carefully inspected, and that is as it should be. Couples are not coerced either into terminating pregnancies or carrying them to term. However, it is possible to imagine this changing. The most likely change is legislation at the state or federal level that would consider fetuses with chromosomal or metabolic anomalies to be protected by the fourteenth amendment (due process and equal protection clauses) and by statutes that prohibit discrimination against the handicapped. In the current climate, it is possible to imagine both the passage of such legislation and its support by rubrics and rhetorics that speak to the state's interest in preserving life. The tragedy here is not just of choice denied, although I do not with to minimize this. There is also the tragedy of having been coerced by the state into having a child with special needs and finding the state unable to provide the basic social supports that such children inevitably require. Such a scenario is all too likely, given the success that pro-life advocates have had at eroding the edges of the right to choice.

Alternatively, it is possible but more difficult to imagine that the state may coerce couples with certain designated positive findings from amniocentesis into abortions. After all, the resource-allocation problems of the welfare state are well documented. The high cost of medical services is well known, and the need for cost-containment is a priority in health care. Tremendous savings could be realized by preventing the births of defective fetuses. It is these savings and the considerable savings in emotional wear and tear that genetic counselors have used to sell their services as a public health measure. In this second scenario, all that changes is the locus of control, the key decision maker. Of course, this is not a small change. Either scenario, coerced childbirth or coerced abortion, is repugnant to the fundamental value of privacy as a cherished element of personhood. But either measure could find support in competing values, either the value of human life or the equitable use of scarce resources. What makes the practice of applied human genetics acceptable is the high degree of individual choice that appears to be exercised. What is left unappreciated is how fragile that choice might be.

A second covert danger in the practice of genetic counseling concerns the level of support open to those born with preventable diseases. It is quite possible that such individuals will be given even less than the niggardly support currently provided. The parents of such children might be viewed as having brought their problems on themselves. Societal tolerance, not so great to begin with, might shrink as the burdens of birth defects become associated with parental neglect in seeking appropriate prenatal care.

It is possible that such a turn of events might not come to pass. Legal protections prevent many of the more overt forms of discrimination against the handicapped and mandate special services, even if adequate funding is a chronic problem. Further, through organized political interest groups, the interests of many of those with genetic defects are advanced. Nonetheless, some erosion of sympathy for those afflicted with genetic disorders may occur, heightened by prevailing doctrines of health puritanism that stress individual responsibility for health outcomes.

Ultimately, the genetic counselors' strategy of treating all of the troublesome questions that crossed their doorstep as private issues worked well to avoid controversy at Nightingale at the time. Genetic counseling, like many other practices, is acceptable because it occurs among consenting adults; however, how long this can continue to be the case is problematic. Further, in treating users of their service the genetic counselors often behave as if all the troublesome issues raised by the application of genetic knowledge have been resolved in other arenas. This is clearly not the case.

Beyond that, some of the most thorny issues raised by advances in genetic knowledge have very little to do with individual consent and the doctor-patient relationship. Genetic fingerprinting—the identification of individuals by their unique genetic makeup—has many forensic applications but also raises considerable questions about civil liberties. Or let us assume a treatment *in utero* to correct a genetic defect. Now consider the difficulties of application. There are the normal questions about cost and allocation, but to those complications we need to add one more. Exactly what is being fixed? Just as the map is not the territory named, genetic makeup is not the person. Treatments *in utero* promise to fix what is broken only in theory. At the very least, they raise questions about how activist and interventionist we wish health care to be. But these are not the only treatments to raise such questions. I found them because I studied genetic counselors; had I studied oncologists, I would have found others.

To continue this line of thought just a bit further, as our mapping of the human genome gets more and more sophisticated, no doubt we will identify the genetic basis of many conditions which are multifactorial, of which genetics is just a part. When this happens, what then? At the moment, the results of amniocentesis when positive are a "bright light" test for future severe deficits. But this will not always be the case; as the biological research grows more sophisticated, positive results will be more equivocal. Already this is so for certain conditions, such as fragile X syndrome, where not everyone with the genetic marker is affected in terms of everyday performance.

The point here is that there is a great deal of truth to Trancredi and Nelkin's (1989) contention that genetics is a dangerous form of diagnostics. The dangers are multiple. On the one hand, they lead us to an increasingly individualistic conception of disease and disability: With careful enough screening, we can eliminate imperfection. The emphasis on genetics as the key to understanding both individuals and individual differences obscures the role that social conditions play in all of this. We can screen for individuals susceptible to toxic substances, or we can eliminate the substances. We can screen to rid the society of those with chromosomal abnormalities, or we can provide decent supportive services for them that make their lives more rewarding and less burdensome to others. Genetic screening is presented as the least costly strategy, but it is not clear that this is so, especially if we factor in how this hypertrophic emphasis on individual causation weakens our collective concern for one another. On the other hand, applied genetics presents to us all a false image of predestined perfectibility. It loosens somewhat our own sense of responsibility for ourselves and what we become.

At any rate, issues of this kind are not engaged in genetic counseling. Indeed it would be odd if they were. This does not mean, however, that they are not real, that they do not need attending to. The problem is, of course, that we have not yet found a convenient forum for discussing these issues. Like Samuels, we may get to the point where we "just want to clone the good people." Before we do, however, we need to consider the cost to us all—and we need to develop more than just an economic definition of cost.

6

AUTONOMY'S END: TOWARD THE FUTURE

All ethnography is a collection of incidents, stories from everyday life, presented in the service of furthering some more general perspective about some aspect of social life—here, the nature of professional service in applied human genetics. As a practical matter, it is difficult to talk with precision about categories of situations, types of behavior, or the rationalization of motives for the universalized and generalized nature of "professional service" on the basis of a case study, no matter how careful we are. However forceful this book's claims about the nature of professional service, they are limited by method. The sample—a single unit in a single hospital—has no greater power than the n of 1 squared. The sample is not adequate, either for describing genetic counselors as members of a profession or as workers in an organization.

Staying strictly in the "bounded whole" of Nightingale Children's Center, I have produced miniaturized descriptions and characterizations of "genetic counselors' work activity" as I happened to be able to observe it. But to what end? The new theoretical freight—the real contribution—is modest. I describe genetic counselors as "tinkering tradespersons" in the pediatric hospitals who fulfill needs which are peripheral to the organization's main mission.

The overarching narrative themes are that (1) rationalization trivializes mystery; (2) service is defined through scientific/technical standards, and (3) affect is funneled out of the hospital. Stated alternatively, with some qualifications this second time, in a hospital encounter, organized around a prenatal diagnosis or a neonate with significant birth anomaly, the genetic counselor in providing service invariably and inevitably depersonalizes, trivializes, or dissolves the meaning of momentous moments in everyday life; or as Hughes would have stated it, the emergencies of lay persons are transformed in the routines of professionals.

There is not much new in this. Close watchers of reproduction and of death and dying have been saying this for quite some time. Moreover, time has rendered much of this narrative quaint—picaresque descriptions of academic clinical medicine in some enchanted domain before the current array of third parties established their place at the bedside. I have produced the equivalent of a once-upon-a-time tale: a description of genetic counseling as hospital work before ethical concern established its formal place at the bedside and during a time when reductionistic genetic thinking was less attractive to policy makers than it is now.

All ethnography becomes social history—a report from the field concerning some recurrent problems of the human condition, indexed in this account by how the natives at Nightingale use such terms as *accident, rare event, mystery,* or *tragedy,* and the shared ways these same narratives developed for explaining, managing, and understanding them. Ethnography also marks a specific moment: the problems it discusses testify to a shared, lived experience with a group of natives somewhere. The ethnographic descriptions of inpatient and outpatient care involving the genetics unit are descriptions of health care which I observed in the past, before the formation of hospital ethics committees, prospective payments, vigorous third-party oversight, Baby M and increasing judicial attention to private commercial surrogacy, Nancy Cruzan and the right to die, public recognition of the need for health-care rationing, the appearance of AIDS, and awareness of the medically indigent. It strikes me that this way of presenting events over a decade old is unfair to my natives. It does not report on the changes they have made with the times.

In this ethnography, the natives somewhere who are being portrayed so unfairly are the genetic counselors of Nightingale Children's Center. They provide the details for instant generalizations about medicine, the professions, and the delivery of services in the hospital. I have described genetic counselors as a group with a "professional service" ethos and then tried to relate that ethos to a set of workplace activities, tasks, routines, and emergencies. Genetic counselors provide outpatient and inpatient services; each has its own demands, norms, values, etiquette, and rules—its own behavioral code.

For outpatient clinical care, legitimate requests for service call forth a clear occupational code of conduct which can be expressed as a few behavioral maxims:[1]

Provide correct information to guide rational decision making, but preserve client choice.
Remember that the choice lies with the woman or the couple.
Behave in a value-neutral, nondirective style so as not to usurp the operation of private choice.
Support but do not interfere with the private choice of the woman or a couple.
Do not jump off bridges because a pregnancy is or is not carried to term.
Evaluate decisions in terms of their "comfort." Can everybody live with them?
Talk to the group if a decision is one you can't live with.

Requests for outpatient service that were seen as illegitimate, such as formal involvement with reproductive or marital decisions at the insistence of worried parents, plaintiff's attorneys, or institutional caregivers, called forth a different code of conduct. The genetic counselors no longer had any specific obligations, since the agent raising the question had no specific right to do so in the first place. Even so, the behavior of the genetic counselors did not vary much in the two situations. The bare genetic "facts" of any case exerted obligations all their own. It was never fair to deny to any user of the service whatever well-established scientific truths there were.

On the inpatient side at Nightingale, the rules were different.

1. I do not want to overly burden the text here with my debts to Durkheim concerning the relationship of occupational and civic morality. Moreover, Hughes was not indifferent to Durkheim. To build on him requires a deepening of the connection through an amplification of the meaning; it permits the growth of an intellectual tradition.

Two sets applied: (1) Rules for consulting with attending colleagues who had primary clinical responsibilities, and (2) rules for consulting with residents. The attendings at Nightingale had responsibilities both for deciding who was a "salvageable" infant and for implementing treatment. In consults with them, great deference was given to the expressed desires of colleagues who chose to wear the "green suit" of clinical responsibility. Ironically, the value-neutral, nondirective style that ratified personal choice in the clinic negated those same choices as a possibility in the pediatric hospital. The residents at Nightingale used consults with genetic counselors to orchestrate communication with parents of hospitalized children, to receive "spot" didactic lessons in genetic diagnosis, or to "cover all bases" in the face of an avalanche of unfolding medical disaster and misadventure.

In this chapter we need to move from Nightingale to the wider world. It is a journey of but two steps. The first is to understand how "clinical applications of human genetics" have changed since these observations were made. Most significant here are changes in both scientific capacity and cultural receptivity. The second is to understand the organizational changes in academic medicine brought about by greater administrative supervision at all levels of accountability, by the increased legitimacy of giving voice to "ethical concern," and by the general dispersion of individualized medical authority to teams. The ethnographic description has been written as if Nightingale were the whole world, as if its team were perfect exemplars of genetic counselors everywhere, as if no changes had occurred since the observations were made. I will not account for changes at Nightingale; to do so I would need to return to the field, and the yield would not be worth the effort. How Nightingale has changed is vitally important, but only to a limited community of liability. How the world has changed is of interest to a much broader one. But first we need to represent the work of Nightingale's genetic counselors as a "shopfloor drama."

The Simple Shopfloor Drama: Humbled Professionals

For Hughes, sociological imagination is exercised when the world is described in ways that reverse "conventional sentimentality."

Given the glamour and prestige of genetic research in academic medicine today, we would expect, on the clinical side, a group of proud professionals whose vocabulary for describing their work conveyed some of the Promethean power of expanded technological capabilities. At Nightingale, genetic counselors exercise a Hughesian sociological imagination when they talk about their work. They speak of themselves as "workers" who "mop up" not only the misfortune and tragedy brought on by genetic errors but also by many other more human failings as well. Their case files are a collection of the "normal accidents" of biology and of the organization of the tertiary-care pediatric center. Such misfirings are an inevitable, theoretically predictable, but empirically random property of complex systems (Perrow 1985).

The genetic counselors at Nightingale grudgingly accepted their mop-up work, but not without resistance. They complained about their colleagues' unwillingness to shoulder the load. Targets of criticism included insensitive attendings and reluctant psychiatrists. They also had problems with family, clergy, and neighbors whose clumsy attempts to help or whose reluctance to intervene often exacerbated the situations which needed mopping up. At any rate, it is easy to imagine how the kinds of situations that would lead to a meaningful meeting with a genetic counselor would be those in which "emotional flooding" was an ever-present possibility. In clinic at Nightingale, when such flooding occurred, the clinic coordinator, the "amnio-counselor," and occasionally the ethnographer ("Bosk, would you like to interview the Quiggles? They have a problem which is a good example of the difficulties Quiggles have everywhere.")[2] were often recruited to help with the mop-up.

Genetic counselors were "buffers, cushions, and shock-absorbers." They were utilized by their colleagues as a service for bereaved parents, for genetic counselors provide a version of what went wrong the last time and what the risks would be the next time to couples whose children were born with significant anomalies. Local pediatricians in the hospital and the community used them as

2. The Quiggle family should be familiar to sociologists who first became aware of their troubles when Erving Goffman (1961b) described in *Stigma* the problems they had with the well-meant but off-the-mark conversational kindnesses offered by strangers.

official labelers of conditions they suspected. Allowing someone else to deliver the bad news was a referral tactic which allowed these pediatricians freedom to focus on the positive in their dealings with the family. Genetic counselors at Nightingale were asked to do a great deal of the dirty "emotions work" that traditionally works its way down the prestige ladder in medicine.

The genetic counselors' vocabulary for describing their work is modest: they perform "song-and-dance routines" for those who visit the clinic. Occasionally, sessions are more stressful, and genetic counselors then liken routines to the magical acrobatics of "walking on eggshells." Even so, the genetic counselors recognize that in the scheme of things, such emotional work does not have very high status at a place like Nightingale. Counseling is not doing, and at places like Nightingale, doing is more esteemed.

There is an active quality to what genetic counselors do *not* do. They do not tell their clients what to do. There is an aspect of protection in this: their passivity is in the service of the client's autonomy. They are value-neutral and nondirective with clients so as to preserve their reproductive rights. This championing of lay autonomy is limited to outpatient services. With their colleagues at Nightingale Children's Center, they take an equally nondirective, value-neutral posture. It is not for them to challenge their colleagues who "wear green suits" unless they are willing to don such a uniform themselves. Genetic counselors only rarely venture so much as the innocent question. They are never forceful advocates of the autonomy of the patients for whom their colleagues have inpatient responsibilities.

The genetic counselors' preservation of the clients' right to private, autonomous reproductive decision making at Nightingale Children's Center was conditioned more by the nature of therapy for birth defects discovered prenatally—second-trimester abortion—than any other factor. Their reluctance to disrupt "green-suited" authority was conditioned by their distance from the day-to-day activities of the wards, from the daily pursuit of care and cure. With the decline of clinical impotence in human genetics, we need to ask, Will outpatient autonomy continue to be defended? Will inpatient autonomy continue to be abrogated? Will genetic counseling remain humble work in a proud place?

A More Complex Reality

In a field of genetic counseling, there has been for some time a movement away from humble role definitions. After all, there are considerable limitations built into any definition of *help* that stresses its delivery in a "value-neutral, nondirective" way. The experience of genetic counselors working in clinics, both at Nightingale and elsewhere, made them well aware of these limitations. As a result, they have adapted and changed. These changes were apparent while I was still in the field. Service is defined more broadly as a result; there is more movement away from "providing correct technical information" as a solitary core task in the definition of professional service. Kessler (1980) argues that a "paradigm shift" has occurred in genetic counseling. The result of this shift is that counselor pay closer attention to the emotional and psychological aspects of client problems. In Kessler' terms, Nightingale is just one center where this shift had not yet taken place, a center, whatever its virtues, that was outside the mainstream.

Actually, the reality was more complex. Among the striking things about the genetic counselors at Nightingale was their ability to recognize the emotional needs of patients and their attempt to meet them, even if in a clumsy way. Value-neutral and nondirective as they were, the genetic counselors occasionally made claims to be practicing within Kessler's psychological paradigm. Their performance was, however, restricted by the typical, one-visit format. The value-neutral, nondirective style, which encouraged clients to state an agenda, allowed genuine issues to emerge. The emphasis on providing correct information as the core task in genetic counseling meant that these genuine issues were simultaneously identified, acknowledged, and ignored.

Twiss (1979) also argues against the limitations imposed by a purely "technical" definition of service: if an adequate service is provided, genetic counselors cannot shirk their responsibilities as moral advisors. For Twiss, moral advice is part of the professional territory of genetic counseling, a domain of expertise, the art rather than the science of professional practice. The genetic counselors at Nightingale preferred the science of genetics to the art of its practice. But practice they did, because this at least assured responsible information. The genetic counselors at Nightingale saw themselves as moral advisers, with advice taking the form of impersonal risk statements. Moral advisors, certainly—but moral advice was reduced to technically correct, scientifically current information.

Advising is different from decision making; each task lodges autonomy with different actors. Reasonable claims about acting as a moral advisor are easily reconciled with a professional minimalism. Anything more than such minimalism threatens to obtrude on clients' privacy and trample upon a couple's or woman's private reproductive rights. The reproductive rights of women are threatened from many directions; it is fair to say that the genetic counselors at Nightingale are not one of the them, nor are they likely to be.

In addition to the psychological and moral-advisor paradigms for characterizing the proper work of genetic counselors, we find a third in the literature. Antley (1979) argues that the genetic counselor's responsibilities as a "decision-facilitator" supersede any obligation to a specific behavioral style. There is a job to be done after all; skill is using tools appropriate for the job. The genetic counselors are and see themselves as "decision-facilitators." But they perform differently than Antley's role-description suggests. For them, skill was not an appropriate choice from a repertoire but success at manipulating a "nondirective, value-neutral" approach. The practice of sending follow-up letters summarizing discussions that may not have been understood to begin with underscores the genetic counselors' faith that objective information delivered in a straightforward manner facilitates decision.[3] Psychological and moral advising, as well as decision-facilitating, are role ideals which can easily accommodate a value-neutral, nondirective professional ethos and style.

Yarborough, Scott, and Dixon (1989) provide recent indirect evidence that a nondirective, value-neutral work ethos of professional service is neither limited to Nightingale, nor entirely outdated. Why else develop an elaborate argument that the push of autonomy be balanced by the pull of beneficence? Why else worry about what

---

3. It is also sound risk management, but that is a story for a different day. For the beginning of that story, see Bosk (1991).

save provide information a genetic counselor must do in order to provide a professional service? It is clear from the appearance of such articles that there is considerable ferment in the field about how genetic counselors should counsel those who use their services, that there is at times an intense tension between the goal of "doing good" and that of "preserving the patient's autonomy." Yarborough, Scott, and Dixon suggest that "humble" genetic counselors overly respectful of client autonomy can fail to act with beneficence. Such false humility in the professional workplace is the equivalent of paternalistic denial of paternalism; it is self-defeating piety.

The three alternative paradigms and their alternative prescriptions for action suggest that the workplace ideology, the professional ethos of genetic counselors, is more varied than I have portrayed it solely by my characterization from Nightingale. Moreover, ample evidence exists from the behavior of the genetic counselors at Nightingale that workplace ideology and professional ethos do not always determine behavior. For while professional commitment to a value-neutral, nondirective style guides practice, it should not be confused with practice. These are professional ideals. Their frequent breaching reminds us of their rare fulfillment. About service provision itself, genetic counselors are not professionally humble; they are not value-neutral and nondirective. Offering services is a way to solve problems. Genetic counselors believe they provide a useful, valuable, cost-effective service to very specific categories of clients. They generally believe in the extension and expansion of the genetic domain as new techniques become available.

Further, value-neutral, nondirective counseling is, like most ideals, easy to espouse but in practice, difficult to perform. At Nightingale such breaches are extremely problematic for the workgroup, yet all members of the group do recognize situations in which service users require more than "just the facts." Exceptions to the nondirective, value-neutral rule are vigorously debated but easily fashioned if needed, or justified if challenged. The essence of professional judgment and discretion is to know when the ordinary rules must be suspended. In the doing, the accountable breaches of the rule or norm are nearly as frequent its successful enactments.

In describing the operation of a value-neutral, nondirective ideology of professional help in genetic counseling, Nightingale Children's Center is not necessarily best-suited to represent the world of clinical practice—Nightingale is just too peculiar for that sort of thing. Nonetheless, the members of the team at Nightingale do not appear radically different from the rest of the profession, according to the descriptive material available. The survey data reported by Sorenson and Cuthbert (1979) and updated and expanded by Wertz and Fletcher (1988, 1989) and Wertz, Fletcher, and Mulvihill (1990) indicate that other American genetic counselors who are M.D.'s or Ph.D.'s share the genetic counselors' underlying work ideology and their flexibility in deploying it, given the circumstances of a particular case. However, Wertz and Fletcher's data indicate that a concern with voluntariness, patient autonomy, and nondirection varies nationally, and a concern with the privacy of an individual's reproductive rights is most fully developed in the American clinical context. American genetic counselors are the most numerous of practitioners, but their attitudes about how genetic knowledge is best applied are not necessarily representative of a more global universe. Nor is the value they place on privacy and confidentiality reassurance that these values will be respected as new genetic technologies develop. After all, they are not a very powerful group. So what is the future for "professional humility" in applications of human genetics?

The Future of Professional Humility

There are two shops in the work of genetic counselors: the laboratory and the clinic, and very different developments are taking place in each. The pace of change of our knowledge base in genetics is breathtaking to behold. Since I left the field, prenatal diagnosis can be done earlier in pregnancy, more conditions can be identified, and genetic cures are spoken of with greater frequency. The emphasis on screening and prevention is giving way to diagnosis and therapy.

Researchers have arrived at a "molecular-level" treatment paradigm to compete with pharmaceutical and surgical therapies. The paradigm rests on precise identification of the genetic material associated with a phenotypic abnormality. The abnormal sequence is removed. A corrected copy of the flawed genetic material is produced and inserted to correct the genotypic mistake. This new material is said to be *inserted, spliced, transplanted, transferred, transcribed,* or *programmed* into the individual. We have not yet gone far down this road, which is parodied above by oversimplification. But the power of this model should not therefore be discounted. Extensions of applied human genetics beyond screening and prevention promise an end to second-trimester abortions premised upon genetic fitness, as well as a reduction in suffering and health-care costs. Unraveling the dynamics of disease at a genetic level holds great promise for many diseases about which much is known but little can be done. Beyond that, the treatments themselves seem less invasive, brutal, and dehumanizing than do therapies currently available in the modern hospital. This is a therapeutic paradigm shift of vast proportion. A veritable revolution in health care is promised with these new treatment technologies. Utopian themes in writing about progress in "applied human genetics" are quite prevalent.[4]

The pace of change in applied human genetics has been accelerated by the Human Genome Project (HGP), which has been described as

> a worldwide research effort with the goal of analyzing the
> structure of the human DNA and determining the
> location of the estimated 100,000 human genes. The
> project, which will cost an estimated $3 billion over
> fifteen years, is widely thought to be one of the most
> important scientific research projects undertaken. It will
> help scientists understand and eventually treat many of
> the more than 4,000 genetic diseases that afflict mankind,
> as well as the many multifactorial diseases in which
> genetic predisposition plays an important part.

4. In fairness, I should note that the standard news release of a genetic breakthrough in the laboratory usually includes, towards the end, a disclaimer of any immediate benefits. If Edgar and Rothman (1990) are right about a relaxation of current regulatory standards, these disclaimers might have to be taken less seriously.

As each part of the human genome is more carefully mapped, as we gain more precise knowledge (the exact implications of which are unclear), and as we verge on cures, we should not expect clinicians/researchers to adopt the nondirective, value-neutral position of genetic counselors. After all, as the HGP description states, it is "scientists," not "physicians" or "counselors," who will employ genetic treatments. The culture of experimental therapy, as the work of Fox (1959), Fox and Swazey (1974), and Kolata (1990) demonstrates, is different. New breakthroughs are more likely to be touted by those who have both developed them and believe in their efficacy than they are to be presented neutrally by information specialists.

Along whatever lines a "new" clinical genetics emerges, genetic counselors will not be leading the way. They lack the ability both to control research breakthroughs and to determine how genetic knowledge is applied outside their own local setting. In the last ten years, the split of bench science and ordinary counseling which Pearl Katz spoke of in Chapter 2 has become more formally articulated in the division of labor.

As the split has grown, so have the ranks in each multiplied. The research side of genetics has prospered both in universities and private industries. One index of the growth of genetics as applied knowledge is the expansion of private enterprises that are developing, marketing, and distributing medical products made available by new genetic technologies.

The growth in the clinical ranks has been less dramatic but no less significant or complex. While the number of genetic counselors providing clinical services has grown, there has also been a change in those who actually provide the service. To the M.D.'s and Ph.D.'s who were clinicians, "accidentally and incidentally," have been added the graduates of postbachelor's programs in genetics. Since the establishment of the program at Sarah Lawrence in 1969–70, fifteen programs have been developed. The American Society of Genetic Counselors now numbers over 1,000. Growth appears assured for a number of reasons.

The field is so young that entrants will outnumber retirees for some time. In addition, the discoveries of the Human Genome Project will create a need for clinical translators. We, our insurance companies, or both are likely to want to know what our genotype "means," regardless of phenotypic variation. This need will be most acutely felt where middle-class rationality and risk-management strategies are most available. But the need is more widely disseminated in the society than that, the prenatal detection of AIDS being no less important than the detection of trisomy 21 or myelomeningocele. In fact, the "need" for genetic counselors is a socially artificial one that depends on a number of variables such as the current state of the art in prediagnostic technology and intervention, the resources and capacities of the best NICUs, public policies toward financing abortion services, the risk-management strategies of obstetrics/gynecology, and other demands on social resources.

But the need for counselors grows also with the capacity to make phenotypic predictions from genotypic evidence. At the very least, obstetric/gynecological services in urban centers need to provide genetic counseling, if only to provide care that can safely be said to meet a community's highest standard of prenatal care. Not to make available such counseling to women facing known risks for preventable defects would surely not be a prudent risk-management strategy for either obstetricians or perinatologists. The need for genetic counseling will grow as well with each new application of genetics to medicine. Each newly discovered "marker" of genetic disease, creates a flood of lab work and a trickle of clinical opportunity.

In the outpatient clinic, to the extent that genetic counselors continue to regard reproductive decisions as private, they will preserve the lay structure of reproductive decision making. In the hospital, it is fair to assume that they will not become forceful advocates of patient autonomy. Here there is no reason to suspect that their collegial deference will be altered because medical ethics has come to the bedside. Nor will the presence of genetic counselors do much to temper aggressive interventions as they become available, in part because patients and parents so often desire them (Zussman 1992).

Autonomy's End: A Committee Decision

It may be that when all is said and done, there is little behavioral change. It is worth remembering, however, how much more needs to be said and done than previously, how all that saying and doing is a change in and of itself, and how much the organizational structure of academic medicine has changed as a result.

Intrainstitutional mechanisms now provide a way for the private agendas of patients and families to be heard alongside the professional ones of medical specialists. Annas (1991) complains that all of these bureaucratic changes may act to co-opt rather than to enhance the patient's experience because those doing the work of ethics take into account the long-run needs of their institutional employers. As a result, rather than a revolution that subserves the rights of lay persons in their encounters with medical authority, we have merely added a layer of institutional protection. We have, thereby, also reduced individual professional responsibility and accountability. In addition, we have confused ethics with conflict between patient and physician, when surely not all that is agreed upon is made ethical by the fact of consensus.

Certainly, when we examine concretely how some specific requirement of care put in place explicitly to magnify patient choice operates, such as new, more muscular understandings of informed consent, we are disappointed (Lidz and Meisel 1984). As we observed them, genetic counselors preserved the autonomy of outpatients and watched silently as it was usurped for inpatients. Moreover, when they most fervently asserted that parents were autonomous, that they had to make their own decisions, the genetic counselors used such a stance to retreat from engaging the emotional issues with which couples struggled. The dark side of patient autonomy was patient abandonment.

Yet it is equally possible that the genetic counselors sheltered couples rather than abandoned them—sheltered them, by providing a place where their private wills could gear into the world without scrutiny. In the long run it is possible that the current clinical bedside, so crowded with strangers and experts, still provides some cover for patients and families to make private decisions appropriate to local circumstances. Localized community decision making protects personal choices.

In the time that I took to learn about genetic counselors, the role that I fashioned for myself—witness—has become formalized as that of the *bioethicist,* and the questions I routinely wished to ask but never did are being incorporated into the delivery of care. Whether patient autonomy and individual rights will increase as a result is, for me, problematic; ethicists who are part of organizations and do not leave them may find themselves not so independent as they wish. Their ability to tell a story may be compromised by their part in the story. There is a call to incorporate ethnography into bioethics, but such an incorporation is hard to imagine. In the current climate, who can claim to be a detached enough observer to provide reliable ethnographic detail?

It is clear that dramatic advances in genetics are upon us. It is also clear that the safeguards—the Institutional Review Boards (IRBs), the bioethicists, the genetic counselors—are not likely to do much to stem the advancing wave of change. It remains to be seen how useful they will be in making sure that change is implemented in sensible ways. Currently, 3 percent of the investment in the Human Genome Project is set aside to explore the likely implications of such advances. We need to do more, or the technically possible will continue to determine the substantively desirable.

7

A TWICE-TOLD TALE
OF WITNESSING

I described earlier how I was invited to join the genetic counseling team, how I thought the invitation carried with it some vague obligation to help, and how I felt that I completely failed to meet that obligation. Then, in a manner surely different from what C. Wright Mills meant when describing sociological imagination, I made of my private troubles a public issue. I indict the genetic counselors for meeting client needs in a perfunctory manner. The fact that their work is anchored in a pediatric hospital allowed me to indict the entire medical profession for its inability to help those with intolerable troubles. I directed my attention to the "rough edge" of practice.

As a result, this account of workplace practices in a pediatric hospital virtually ignores the "smooth interface." I entirely fail to mention, or mention only in passing, that the limited goals counselors set for themselves—providing the most value-neutral assessment of conditional probabilities—was often what the person asking the question most wanted, whether that person was a treating physician or a lay service user. Rather than parading the countless examples of those occasions where genetic counseling, or the overall medical care of which it is but a small part, is a triumph of expectations fulfilled, I carefully dissect those occasions when genetic counselors, or others in the pediatric hospital where they worked, found themselves frenetically navigating a situationally stormy rough edge. Few if any "smooth interfaces" get displayed in typography that signals their status as relics from my fieldwork note-books.

When the genetic counselors invited me to study them, it was with the expectation that I would produce a portrait, "warts and all." With ethnographic license, I produced one that looked only at warts. I have always assumed that such one-sided attention was necessary to construct ideal typical accounts of social process in bounded wholes, which is what I take the task of ethnography to be. With full ethnographic faith and self-confidence, I paid less attention to the fact that more than a single one-sided account is possible, or that my one-sided account might be unfairly distorted.

After all, a quite different account is possible. The genetic counselors could be just as easily described as heroic individuals able to suppress their own preferences and provide value-neutral statements of conditional probabilities. As experts, they do not let their values intrude on their professional/technical expertise. Approaches to care such as the counselors adopt reverse professional dominance in dealing with clients and avoid intraprofessional wrangling in the workplace when dealing with colleagues. Certainly the restraint of genetic counselors in the service of patient autonomy deserves more credit than it is given in the text.

There is another alternative. The genetic counselors are only "occasional" clinicians. Their limited patient-contact hours and responsibilities free them to meet research obligations and allow them to meet the demands of family life or pursue personal interests. The organizational niche of genetic counselors could have been presented as an attractive solution to the tension between the "greedy" claims of the service obligation and those of self, family, and community (Coser 1974). The boundaries that genetic counselors place around their involvement in clinical activity could have been presented as an ingenious tactic for preserving a personal self in a professional occupation (Zerubaval 1979; Broadhead 1983; Gerber 1983).

I also never stopped to worry that some of the data might have been gathered unethically. After all, I sometimes lacked fully informed, voluntary consent. While genetic counselors volunteered for study, other pediatricians were observed without their knowledge, as were patients; when consulting, there sometimes was not ample opportunity to introduce the ethnographer. If opportunity existed, it was hard to imagine at the time how the introduction would help a troubled situation.

Two instances of ethnography without consent are prominently displayed and analyzed in the text. Neither Doctor Marceau nor the Doughertys (Chapter 3) had any idea who I was as I sat next to Bill while they had their options conference. I note in my description that Bill is angry at Marceau but fails to say anything. Like Bill I was angry too. I sat silent as a stump. A question from me would surely have remedied the defect in care that the text complains of. How can I tell this story now about "using didge and diuretics to let nature take its course" if it fails the most basic ethical muster for research? This is guilty knowledge. Is their any benefit to telling the story? Could there be any harm?

I also lacked fully informed, voluntary consent in both Baby Doe cases, though in slightly different ways. I had an open invitation to attend weekly clinical genetics rounds. The first day I attended was the day that "the baby" in chapter 4 was discussed. People spoke freely and learned later that a witness was recording their words. In the second case, I was someone who came to a conference about a case whose management had troubled the pediatric staff. The purpose of the meeting was to air those differences and leave them behind. In such meetings, the ethnographer retrieves what the workgroup wishes buried. I was at a public meeting at which the public understanding was that there would be no public record. I have created one. Did I have the right to do that? Does the hiatus in time between collection and the breach of confidentiality mitigate at all the absence of consent? Does consent matter in ethnography? How?

In this chapter, I want to return to my self-casting as a witness, but this time in terms of tensions I felt as I collected data. I want to re-capture the decisions I made along the way about what to observe, what to notice, and what to present. In addition, since I located my analysis in my own sense of powerlessness when called upon by the genetic counselors to help, I need to describe here those situations in which the counselors asked for help and how I helped them or let them down.

Ethnography and Editing

Ethnography is an immensely selective description of social life. What we observe is always less than what happened; what our notes record is always less than we observe; what a book includes is always but the merest fraction of notes. Ethnographers need to analyze the materials they include in their accounts and need as well to say something of what they exclude.

Chapters 2 through 5 of this text concentrate on formal meetings between physicians and parents or among physicians and other health-care professionals. Almost everything reported in the text occurs in an arena, or is an activity that has a formal name in the pediatric hospital. This is much more an account of what people did in public situations than what they privately felt about them. Where the text recounts private feelings, it generally reports on their expression in professional arenas (such as postclinic conferences) expressly created for the purpose of airing those sentiments. The stress on professionally public arenas was one way for me to resolve both the objectivity and the consent problem. Even so, the ethnographic practice of using the best notes, the most dramatic cases, the most floridly described situations undermines the objectivity sought. Moreover, the ethnographic selection from fragments is inherently problematic, since the same fragments can be arranged into so many other alternative accounts. Beyond that, a multiplicity of alternative accounts lie buried in field materials not cited.

Fieldnotes are representative, but ethnographers choose what it is they represent. At any rate, there is an inherent tension between an objective, empirical, ethnographic description and sociological frames of reference committed to examining the rough edge, reversing conventional sentimentality, or more simply describing the "contestable" autonomy of parents, prospective parents, and physicians.

The fieldworker can do more, however, than formally describe an ethnographic database, a set of self-generated fieldnotes, and the principles by which they were manipulated. The ethnographer can try to explain what is no longer stored in the notes or memory, what is not available for latter analytic working over. Ethnographers like me have trouble enough making sense of what is in our notes. We are often overwhelmed by the intricacy of what we observed. But—the point warrants repetition—we need to think as well about what we did not see, or what we saw but omitted from our fieldnotes. If we let our data speak to us and only report what happened, there is much that an interpretative ethnographic account cannot offer. Structured silences[1] and baffling omissions are important. We have to learn to identify and interpret them.

Structured Silence in Fieldnotes

One active way I have found for doing this is by encouraging those I observe to repair the silences that I notice and consider proper to ask about. I record both what the genetic counselors did and said and a great deal of their commentary on actions not taken. In my notes, there is a continuing conversation, mostly with Bill, but with all the others as well—a conversation made out of my asking someone why they had done one thing rather than another. After a while in the field, the genetic counselors volunteered such explanations without my asking. In a spontaneous burst of talk, they would formally articulate their decision tree. I assume that all ethnographers have such conversations with subjects. We teach by our questions what we are interested in; our subjects learn what we are interested in and volunteer answers to questions unasked. Such questions are the fieldworker's equivalent to the genetic counselor's passing parents a karyotype: they are a knowledge template.

We explicitly ask about the structured silences and the baffling omissions of others. But what of our own? I found my fieldnotes empty in three places where I expected them to be rich with data. These are worthy of description and analysis.

Closet Conferences

The text reports that the Delberts' (the couple with possible G-syndrome) counseling session was interrupted. I noted that such interruptions were frequent and marked for me how genetic coun-

---

1. I am grateful to my colleague Renée Fox for the term.

selors failed to provide, at a basic level, any counseling at all. I did not note, but probably should have, that the work team on clinic day viewed such interruptions very differently.

For them, they provided opportunities to help in "story repair" when proper examination exploded understandings arrived at during rounds, for gathering composure after a patient dropped a "bombshell" in a session,[2] for figuring out what to do with the unexpected couple who just showed up or with the edgy couple waiting with justifiable impatience for the colleague who had not yet appeared. The Delberts' interruption was one of the few times that I did not excuse myself and go with Smith, Samuels, or Giordano.[3] That fact explains why it is recorded in my notes. When I left, I didn't record it. So, although I am sure such interruptions were "frequent," I cannot prove it with the kind of evidence that I have learned to trust; it's not recorded in my fieldnotes.

One of the reasons that I am sure such interruptions happened frequently is that I remember so vividly where the impromptu consultations arranged at the price of interruptions occurred: the supply closet, which was really a treatment room too small for conducting an examination. I remember being frequently huddled in the closet with the group. But this is not in my notes either. Moreover, closet conversations were more frequent than interruptions. They could occur legitimately between scheduled appointments, before work began, and as it ended, before the fully assembled group trooped over to the official conference room in an adjoining part of the hospital.

Why are the meetings in this space never recorded? The omission is even more startling in an ethnography that claims expressly some linkage to the work of Hughes and his students. After all, the supply closet is the quintessential backstage as described by Hughes's student, Erving Goffman:

> Here the team can run through its performance, checking
> for offending expressions when no audience is present to

2. An example would be the surprise announcement of pregnancy by a couple with very real risks.

3. If Berger were present, no interruptions were brooked. Berger considered them "unprofessional." My notes record few times when Palmer's cases were counseled at the genetics clinic.

be affronted by them; here poor members of the team
who are expressively inept can be schooled or dropped
from the performance. Here the performer can relax, he
can drop his front, forget speaking lines, and step out of
character. (1959, 112)

Ethnography is prized over other methods for its ability to go
beyond understanding formal staged performances; it reveals the
grimier backstage arrangements necessary for formal staging. It is
the backstage that is the repository of prized knowledge about how
workers feel about their work, how they understand what they are
doing, and how the define what the right thing to do is, in any situation. Yet my notes are empty of closeted information. Why? I knew
the conversations were important. How do I excuse their omission
first from my consideration and then the reader's?

As a sociologist, it easy here to fall into some variant of ecological
determinism. Spatial arrangements made it impossible. It was a
small supply closet; that smallness made unobtrusive note-taking
impossible. This tidy explanation overlooks the routine writing
others did in the supply closet and the fact that I had no qualms
about the obtrusiveness of my note-taking in counseling sessions,
where I scribbled furiously as genetic counselors and parents
talked. In any case, not taking notes at the time does not explain
why there is no mention in my notes of these conferences. Quite a
lot makes its way into my fieldnotes that I do not write down at the
time. As an ethnographer, I take some justifiable pride in my ability
to recall insignificant details. So how could the workgroup's most
routinized backstage activity fall out of this account?

This is partly a matter of manners. One of the first times that I
participated in a closet conference, I was told and asked, "This kind
of discussion has nothing to do with what you're studying, right?" I
remember being evasive; offering reassurance but fully intending
to gather as much of "that kind of discussion" as I could. But I did
not. The genetic counseling group set some observational boundaries; as best I understood them, I tried to respect them. Subjects
have privacy rights, determining their exact nature is difficult to do
with precision.

Where this account provides backstage performances—Bill

and Al's disagreement over who "wears the green suit" or the team's discussion of when patient decisions give one cause "to jump off a bridge"—I have breached that boundary despite notes that are the model of restraint. Keeping "supply-closet conferences" out of them is an index of that restraint.

BERGER'S DEPARTURE

The second structured silence of my notes involves Berger's passing from and Palmer's coming to the workgroup. One would think that such change in leadership would be a natural topic for a workplace ethnography. Berger was a figure who linked the "old" and the "new" Nightingale Children's Center. Nationally, Nightingale's standing in clinical genetics was clear: it was "Berger's shop." His departure itself was an early indicator of the passing of the first post–World War II generation of physicians from academic pediatrics. Berger had a general pediatrics practice, albeit a small one, as well as his counseling cases. He was a representative of the last group of individuals able to link the clinical side and the bench science. None of the others who acted as genetic counselors maintained any general pediatrics caseload, although Giordano maintained a large high-risk obstetrics practice. Berger's departure is an example of the growing distance between general and specialty practice at Nightingale Children's Center and other hospitals of its eminence nationally, as well as an indicator of how genetic counseling services were becoming part of standard obstetrical care.

But there is precious little of Berger's departure in my notes. In fact, my notes from the time Berger announced his departure until Palmer clearly had assumed his duties display a number of odd characteristics. First, the notes from this period are almost exclusively of who said what in counseling sessions or discussion of cases from conferences. Little talk that is off-track is noted. Second, the notes themselves are somewhat more spare and unelaborated than notes taken earlier or later. For example, couples are very rarely described or even named, beyond "the couple." There is a remote mechanical feeling in all of the notes taken at this time. In addition, during the time of Berger's leaving, I made myself generally available to the work group. In fact, I had some need to be around them to listen and to talk. Berger was my patron too, in a loose manner of speaking—if not my patron, my elder. In the local community I grew up in, that counted for something.

So it was not the case that the genetic counselors did not talk about Berger's departure, nor that I made myself so scarce that I never heard them. In fact, I remember long talks within the group as a whole and with each individual about it. But Berger, with his invitation, had set a mandate: I was asked to study the problems of providing genetic counseling as a service. Clearly, the problems caused by personnel changes at Nightingale Children's Center and their consequences for health care were well outside that mandate.

THE PATIENT'S PERSPECTIVE

The third structured silence in my notes, unlike the other two, has nothing to do with my reverence for the sensitivities of those I observed. It has much more to do with the feeling that I could never shake that there was something mildly goulish about the inquiry I was conducting. The last structured silence in my notes involves the patient's perspective. I did not try to enter the patient's perspective as completely as I did with physicians.

During the "pilot" part of this research, Smith, Giordano, or Samuels asked the counselees if they minded "if other members of the group joined us for today's session." No "users of the service" ever said no. The genetics counselors exercised some censorship, steering me away from cases that were "inappropriate for an observer." Of course, those cases intrigued me the most. When the pilot project ended, a consent form was given to all those who came to clinic whom I was scheduled to observe. But the consent form did not hamper cooperation either. Only one person ever refused to participate in the study. She was right to refuse; she should never have been asked.

My notes do not record whether she was asked at my insistence over the genetic counselor's objection, or whether we were a collusive net—they might have wanted me to watch Samuels work. (The woman felt that her albinism caused others to think of her as "a freak.") As Samuels recounted the case, I remember thinking,

"There's no way that that session would have gone as well had I been there."

This was a jolting realization, as was its logical extension that perhaps much of my critique of genetic counseling is nothing more than an index of the strength of observer effect. Perhaps the kind of candid dialogue between genetic counselors and their clients which I find missing is missing because no one talks like that in front of a stranger, an intruder into the meeting with the genetic counselors.

I did make some feeble efforts to understand the parents' point of view in greater depth. For a number of parents, I conducted formal interviews. I use some of this material in the text; but I never really learned to talk with parents, to draw them out. I was not comfortable listening to the details of their pain. When the study began, I did not have children; I was deaf to the meaning of the parents' stories. When I became a parent, I tuned out the parents. It was simply too terrifying for me to try to place myself in their shoes.

I had opportunities to become more involved that I declined. The couple whose husband had been exposed to Agent Orange tried to recruit me for some advocacy work. I declined, but only after I turned off the tape recorder and explored for a while what they wanted. Had I accepted, I might have become the kind of "maverick" that Brown and Mikkelson (1990) say is so necessary to get environmental influences noticed in the public arena. Another time, a couple who had come in for what the text speaks of as "routine bereavement counseling" (their child had died from Sudden Infant Death syndrome, and they were seeking reassurance that its cause was not genetic) invited me to come to their support group to see more closely how parents come to terms with grief. Again I declined.

On the genetic counseling side, Nancy Thomas had made an effort to get me interested in the support groups that are organized around specific genetic conditions. I have a folder full of the *Trisomy 13/18 Newsletter*. It is full of proud parental letters, helpful hints and advice, and reporting of birthdays. The folder is one research lead never fully explored, never fully integrated into the analysis. Finally, I never responded to the urging of another genetic counselor at an institution other than Nightingale that I carefully observe a third genetic counselor at yet another institution who worked closely with patient advocacy groups—a role eschewed by the genetic counselors at Nightingale, but nonetheless an important one for medical professionals and an interesting one to medical sociologists.

Of course, some closer contact with parents was unavoidable. Asking if I might interview them, then probing them about the experience of having a child die, or their understanding of the genetics, or poking around for evidence of discord in families felt intrusive, especially without a previous relationship and no promise of a continued one. With parents, I tended to be a "sociologist collecting data" rather than a person talking to other people. This is not a research style I recommend, although it served my emotional needs well. I shielded myself from parents with an extraordinary amount of formal pretense, but there were some who occasionally broke through to me anyway:

> I had asked the Cranshaws if I might interview them. They had already signed a consent form. They asked what I was going to do with the interview. I said I would answer but asked why they asked. Mrs. Cranshaw said: "Well, if someone comes in and starts asking questions, you want to know who they are, and you wonder why he wants to know these things. I mean, I thought maybe you're writing a book. I admitted as much, and Mrs. Cranshaw replied: "Alright, so we're kind of going to be exploited."

These were my sentiments exactly. I had trouble concentrating during the rest of the interview as they told the story of their child's death. Instead, I kept asking myself to what end did I choose to do this. My most persistent memory of parent interviews is of myself as a polite, soft-spoken, psychological terrorist, whose questions abraded the thin tissue of cover parents had been able to place between themselves and great pain. Moreover, this tissue was one which the genetic counselors treated with great delicacy. It was almost as if my interviews somehow violated the "informal working" procedures of the group I was studying.

I did not like doing this fieldwork. But beyond that, I wondered how Bill Smith and Al Samuels survived in a clinical context in which they saw routinely so much horror and had so few opportunities for clinical "coups" (Bosk and Frader 1990). Joe Giordano, at least, had the compensating heroics of his high-risk obstetric practice. But for Bill and Al, the positives were tragedy averted, which, while it is an accomplishment, is not one without its darker side. I remember once asking Bill how he functioned in the Nightingale environment, how he came to grips with all the "accidents" or "mistakes" that he saw.

> What you have to do is this, Bosk. When you get up in the
> morning, pretend your car is a spaceship. Tell yourself
> you are going to visit another planet. You say, "On that
> planet terrible things happen, but they don't happen on
> my planet. They only happen on that planet I take my
> spaceship to each morning."

I never got as good as Bill at spaceship travel, at seeing Nightingale as another planet. I never mastered the language of its people. One of the few things that ethnography can do is represent those who would otherwise go unrepresented in collective debate. I have failed to do this for those on the other side of the counseling relationship.

In earlier fieldwork, looking at moral agency and general surgery residents and attending faculty, I likewise ignored the patient perspective (Bosk 1979). There, where the patient was anesthetized on the table, ignoring the patient did not make much of a difference. In the context of genetic counseling, where decision-making responsibility rests not with genetic counselors but with parents, or is contested because parents are thought to be tainted fiduciaries for their children's "best interests," this exclusive focus on medical professionals is more problematic, if only because moral agency is so much more complex.

I claim to have been a witness to the work of genetic counselors at Nightingale Children's Center, but this "witnessing" seems oddly pitched. I was so much a participant in some aspects of the genetic counselors' work that I never stepped back and took notes on them. But closet conferences were fundamental to understanding how the workers understood their work. Further, at a time—the transition from Berger to Palmer—when the meaning and nature of the work was being openly reappraised, and when the genetic counselors told me something that was, as Bill would put it "not for public consumption," or as Al, Joe, Mary, and Nancy might say "not . . . the kind of thing I would say publicly," I censored my notes for them. But how and why? Such material—background understandings and backstage performances—are central to ethnographic portraits of professional workplaces. In addition, a deep engagement with the point of view of the user of genetic services was something I assiduously avoided. In effect, I am silent as a witness on those matters where as an ethnographer, I might be expected to write most forcefully.

Beyond that, is there not something hypocritical in trying to wrap these observations with a Hughesian cloth? The words are there, the proper incantatory formulas—"dirty work and good people," "routines and emergencies," "the rough edge of professional practice," and "guilt-sharing and risk-spreading devices"—but the spirit is all wrong. I shunned the humble and hung with the proud. And I was never properly "unconventionally sentimental" (Becker 1970) with them.

Intimacy and Distance

While I was in the field gathering data, I heard Hughes comment on a paper ("If Simmel Were a Fieldworker") presented by Eviatar Zerubavel (1979). Hughes, who was in the audience, suggested that the title was misleading, that Simmel was an extraordinary fieldworker, a cataloger of the variety in "the intersection of social circles." One type that Simmel draws with some care is "the stranger."

The stranger, as Simmel describes him, confronts, like the ethnographer, the "particular constituents and partisan dispositions of the group" with a distinctly "objective attitude." But that objectivity is quickly tested in the field. As Simmel notes, the stranger "who moves on . . . receives the most surprising revelations and confidences, at times reminiscent of a confessional, about matters which are carefully hidden from everybody with whom one is close."

Ethnographers enter the field as strangers, but they cannot remain strangers long, and they do not move on so quickly. Gathering data on a group's ongoing life by observations means entering the group's workplace. For me, this has always involved requests from the workgroup for help. Surgeons (1979) asked me to push chart racks, open "four-by-fours," or "shine that light over here." What I was asked to do rarely disturbed what I was watching. An exchange took place; they let me hang around, but I had to give menial help back. Menial help was always welcome. There was always more than enough scut work to do.

Genetic counselors also asked me to help, but the help requested was no longer so trivial. It very often involved serious professional business: "Talk to this couple for a while and see if you can get a fix on them"; "Watch Al handle this case, and make sure he doesn't steamroll the patients"; "Observe Berger because we are worried about what he is going to say." I never questioned the legitimacy of any of these requests, perhaps seduced by the idea that I had something valuable to offer in a clinical setting, even if I did not precisely know what that something was. The genetic counselors spoke to me as a member of the genetics counseling team; more important, I agreed to listen as a member of the team. How else explain the nearness of being in the supply closet with physicians and the distance of interviewing patients with a formal interview protocol.

To this social distance add the formality of getting a signed consent and audiotaping an interview, and the discontinuities between the ways I know the medical professional's perspective and that of the user of medical services are quite striking. Moreover, I was not a neutral, a "stranger," to the users of service. I was just another white, male doctor in a tie asking questions and taking notes. So my interviews with ordinary lay users of services were not the transcendentally confessional experiences a Simmelian stranger/researcher might hope for.

As a member of the team, I had certain obligations. The first was immersion in team activities. Immersion was not difficult to sustain, since team activity was focused on weekly preclinic rounds, clinic, and postclinic conferences. At other times, Al Samuels was in his lab, Joseph Giordano was at his obstetrics practice, and Bill was on call at Nightingale. At these times, I was released from the yoke of team demands. I taught classes, read, wrote, did committee work—the banal dreary task of ordinary teaching, which corresponded to the clinical banality of genetic counseling.

There was one other weekly gathering at which members of the genetics team were present, but I chose not to attend it. This was the weekly amniocentesis meeting, a Monday-morning case conference chaired by Giordano. At this meeting, the genetic counselors were submerged within a larger obstetrical context in an urban academic teaching hospital. This was defined as an obstetrics rather than a genetics event. I accepted that explanation and stayed away. After all, an ethnographer must observe something rather than everything. Genetic counselors were part of my something; obstetrics was not.

Staying away lowered the demands of the fieldwork. The post-clinic conference ended late afternoon or early evening on Fridays. The amnio conference began at eight on Monday mornings. I could not tolerate the sense of "being captive" that being with the genetic counseling team at the beginning and end of each work week created. Had my threshold for contact been higher, I would have been in a better position to observe the ways in which routine genetic counseling was transformed into routine amnio (and now routine chorionic vacilli sampling [CVS]) counseling and how much of the work was absorbed into the ordinary structure of obstetric care.

Besides the obligation of immersion and the obligation to respond to requests for help, the group expected from me a certain amount of loyalty expressed as circumspection. This should not have been difficult to provide. After all, ethnographic ethics require confidentiality. Simply put, we do not gossip about our subjects, except for our formal presentations and publications. The genetic counselors' demand for loyalty was nothing more than the expectation that I would not tell tales, and as such, it was one common to all ethnography, one I was familiar with as an experienced fieldworker. It was an expectation that was more easily breached than I realized.

When I got to clinic, Bill said he wanted to speak to me about a case. He took me into an examining room and immediately began to talk. He said that he had spoken to my "friend, Farley" and that he had said he had heard that he (Bill) was not too happy with the way the case of a lethal form of dwarfism that they had counseled together had gone. The clear implication here was that I was the one who had told Farley this.

I don't remember telling Farley that. I do remember discussing the case with him. I do remember his being unhappy that the mother of the child had felt that the damaged child was a punishment for an elective abortion that she had had at sixteen. Farley felt that Bill did nothing other than repeat the bare facts of transmission to alleviate the mother's guilt.

I do remember mentioning to Farley that I thought in general that Bill was uncomfortable with expressions of affect in those he counseled. Bill, I said, defined his job as merely disseminating factual information, which he believed would all by itself remove the psychological burdens of genetic defects for parents.

After I spoke to Farley, I asked Bill and Nancy Thomas about the case. They both said that the session had gone terribly. They each described the session as a "classic case" of a woman who was feeling punished for something she had done a long time ago.

I asked them both how they managed these feelings in the session. They mentioned that the pediatrician in the case had suggested that they suggest that the woman talk to her clergyman about it. They said that this was a strategy they avoided until they had an opportunity to "check out" how the clergyman felt about such issues—the last thing they wanted was the guilt being reinforced.

I had thought that I had been particularly skillful in this case at "triangulating," or collecting multiple accounts. Bill, it seemed, now thought less of my practice of my craft. I had trouble listening to Bill, had trouble keeping straight his actual words. I knew he was mad that I had discussed this with Farley. I knew I had been wrong to discuss the case at all with Farley. I was mad at myself. I was mad at Farley for using me to support his evaluation of the handling of the case. I thought he had projected his feelings in the guise of mine. [At any rate, it is one thing to break confidentiality; it is another thing to be found out.]

Bill told me "to be careful, that what happened, it wasn't good." But I already knew that. Then Bill announced, "Well, now it's aired and that's that." And indeed it was, in a way that mirrored the complaint itself. Bill had described what happened; but he did not offer me an opportunity to say my piece, nor had he commented on his feelings. His anger was value-neutral and nondirective.

Then Bill invited me into his next case with him. A gesture, much appreciated, that showed that, despite my indiscretion and his scolding, we were still friends.

To underscore the invitation, he added that the case was "interesting."

"Why?" I asked.

He told me a story about a woman (the person we were about to see, in fact) whose husband had threatened to "kill her and her baby, just last week. The husband had been shipped off to a mental hospital in Florida." Bill presumed the reason for this was that that was where his parents resided.

I agreed that it did "sound interesting." We then negotiated about how interested I was allowed to be. I asked if I could tape the session. "No," said Bill, "it would be too much like giving the woman the third degree." I asked about an interview. "Inappropriate, given the circumstances of the case," said Bill. "What about a consent form," I asked. Again Bill said no. I went along again, not voicing my own objections to this way of doing research.

This is a "confessional tale from the field" (Van Maanen 1988), quoted at great length because it is so instructive of both the strengths and weaknesses of this piece of fieldwork. I think now that I should have had it out with Bill over the consent issue. I believe that the failure to gain a consent was a frequent occurrence, especially when cases were defined as "interesting," but I did not keep a running record of this delict in my field notes. But every time I proceeded without a consent, I compromised the research in important ways.

I think I knew that this was so at the time; my notes indicate a running internal dialogue with myself over the issue, but never an open public one with the group. My hesitancy to do this, which eventually became my failure to do this, I can quite easily rationalize: The research began in a preliminary way, which established ongoing ways of doing things. When a formal consent requirement was instituted, I had already decided to concentrate my attention as a sociological ethnographer on medical professionals and their workplace definitions of proper action. To insist on consent now, when I had been welcomed as a team member, would have jeopardized my access by placing loyalties in question.

Moreover, I was acutely aware of how many researchers before me had tried to study this group and had been actively rebuffed or had decided that this was a game not worth the candle. But I had committed myself to the challenge, not just because I thought the then-practiced clinical applications of genetics were sociologically interesting, but also because I thought the team at Nightingale would allow me access to a range of problematic situations for which ethnographic descriptions would be "good to think with," a way of giving behavioral specificity to a set of "essentially-contestable" concepts like *patient autonomy, treatment decision, private matter, random accident* and *freak occurrence*. The genetic counselors provided me legitimate access to the world of Nightingale. In exchange, I gave up my professional autonomy as a researcher to ask what I wanted of whom I wanted.

Staying away from patients had more or less been a condition of earlier research, so I underestimated its importance in this research. What I had not factored in was that for most patients, only one visit with a genetic counselor was necessary. In another setting, say the intensive care units studied by Guillemin and Holmstrom (1986) or Zussman (1992), the absence of an initial introduction would not have been a fatal flaw. Over time, as patients and families assimilated the culture and procedures of the ICU, the sociological observer was seen simply as one more person with a vague task. While not critical to care or treatment decisions in this setting over time, the ethnographer is available to talk, which has a value all its own.

In genetic counseling, however, my collusion with Bill, my not gaining a consent when that was not only appropriate, but in fact required by a University Institutional Review Board (of which I was a member), shut the lay recipients of genetic counseling services out of the study. After all, having been introduced as a member of the team, I could hardly approach people and explain how what Bill or Al or Joe had said, by way of introduction, "wasn't true," and that "I wasn't really a member of the team," and that "I wanted to ask them about how they really felt and what they really understood about the counseling session."

Further, not having my "outsider" status clarified up front effectively silenced the participant half of this participant observer in two ways. First, couples, if confused, if in need of another opinion, if struggling with the medical professionals of Nightingale Children's Center and in need of an ally, could never turn to me and say "What do you think?" At the time of the fieldwork I thought of this as a benefit. It made me confident that there was little "observer effect," that I had not disturbed the field I had set out to describe, that I had not produced an account of how I stirred the dust striding into the field.

Now, with very great hindsight, it seems to me that more observer effect would have produced more understanding, a deeper appreciation on my part of the experience of the lay users of counseling services. For surely I would have been asked questions by a lay user only as a last resort, after all other alternatives to put together a usable version of reality had failed. At that point, I would have been able to pinpoint with some precision breaches and gaps between professional practices and lay understandings. The words that lay users of genetic services might have addressed to me had they been able, had I an existence and identity apart from "team member," surely would have pointed me toward the "rough edge of practice." It is not hard to imagine that interviews might have been more productive, had I appeared to be less a formal agent of the team.

Beyond that, entering any scene as an "unannounced observer" forced me into silences like the one with Marceau and the Doughertys, which were themselves more unnatural than the dreaded observer effect I so much wanted to avoid. Normally, I think that my own credentials as a student of social life entitle me to "identify group problems and suggest solutions for them," but by not claiming such an identity, I deprived myself of a voice. More a shadow than a witness, I could not transform myself into an ally or advocate. Feeling that I observed under false pretenses, I lacked the right to ask the seemingly innocent question or make the innocuous suggestion that might help a stalled group get from there to here.

When all is said and done, it strikes me as peculiar that at the same time when sociologists were touting clinical skills in organizational and management realms or were retreating from value-neutrality and producing "advocacy ethnography," committed to privileging a particular political perspective, I should fashion such an oddly passive role for myself, one that would neuter my knowledge in this arena of reproductive decision making. I suppose it is quite possible that I was simply mirroring the nondirective ethos and value-neutrality which we have seen were such important parts of the work ideology of genetic counselors, that I overidentified with them so completely that I overgeneralized their workplace ideology, bootlegging it into my discipline from theirs. It is also possible that I was responding to tensions I felt within the discipline of sociology concerning the production of ethnography. By staying silent, by remaining aloof, I was trying to guarantee an objectivity I felt would be shattered by more direct involvement. Finally, I suppose that the "witness" role I fashioned was a "guilt-shifting" and "risk-spreading" device. If I never volunteered suggestions, if I insulated myself from the possibility of being asked the horrible "What would you do?" question, then quite clearly I could not make a mistake. I could not overstep my bounds.

Whatever my motives at the time, I would never again be so passive in a piece of research, I would never again pretend I had so little to offer, I would never again delude myself into thinking that being a "witness" was enough. The next time, the point would not be to describe and interpret the world, but to change it.

And here, as an ethnographer, I am at sea. I do not know how to change it. Moreover, if the point of being in a situation is to improve it through some sort of directed action, which could be as incisive as a scalpel or as gentle as a question, then the activity is no longer "doing ethnography." It is incorrect to say that ethnographers burn out; instead, we become experts in substantive domains. With this expertise and some of its organizational and cultural accoutrements (titles, committee memberships, public forums such as rounds and case conferences) goes some obligation to speak clearly about ongoing cases. My "expert talk" as an ethnographer on a genetic counseling team structured my subject's notion of what I found interesting, what they should tell.

In this case, the genetic counselors talked with me often in a very backstage way; for the users of the service. I was a white, male professional doing "research." I was much too close to one part of the doctor-patient dyad and remote from the other. This caused a regrettable silence at times.

Here, There, and Everywhere

The question of whether to describe pseudonymnously or to correctly identify is both an epistemological and ethical question for ethnographers. To describe pseudonymnously would seem too willful a distortion of a very objective reality. What is more real than the proper names of people and institutions? A second defect of calling someplace real *Nightingale,* and of identifying a specific person with a fictive name is that such accounts of local culture scrub away the very details that make one local culture different from all the rest. If I were more committed to phenomenology, I might say that pseudonyms remove a place's "this-oneness": all those markers which make it unique. Pseudonyms, by the norms of science alone, should be disqualified, since they name both unreliably and unverifiably.

Moreover, the normal conditions that justify pseudonyms do not apply here, as one reviewer of the manuscript pointed out to me. The genetic counselors are not urban outlaws or political revolutionaries whose lives I might somehow endanger if the police or the government read my manuscript. They are physicians and other health professionals in a setting which has received no shortage of discussion. What is to be gained by pretending that "Nightingale" is not somewhere real? Who will be fooled anyway? Generally, pseudonyms are quickly decoded. Everybody soon learns that *Street Corner Society* was done in Boston and that *Experiment Perilous* was done across the river at the Brigham. Why play games? Why insist on Nightingale?

There are a number of reasons. There is, first of all, a question of form. When writing about such mundane matters as the organization of services in a pediatric hospital from the perspective of a team of genetic counselors, to name names is to overspecify. What is important is not the specific person who did something but the less personal rationales that supported the doing. Naming names places the emphasis on the specific and not the general forms of a situation. For journalists (Lukas 1991) and Bauhaus architects, "God may be in the details," but in doing ethnography, a more secular aesthetic prevails.

There is the question of preestablished agreements. One part of the informal, unwritten agreement that was struck to allow me to watch this workgroup so intensely was, "You can report what you want. But you cannot report specifically who and where." On the counselors' part this was a reasonable restriction to make, since it protected patient confidentiality. I assimilated the professional norm of confidentiality in a way that mirrors the text and the world: I distanced myself from service users. For the first summer that I made observations (June 1976), my field notes are ordered by cases identified by service user names. The longer I am in the field, the less frequently are service users identified by name. They all become couples, a she or a he with an occasional baby, girl, or boy. On my part, patient confidentiality was a reasonable thing to assure. I could not see then and I cannot see now why the cast of characters should be properly named.

In fact, I have never understood why anyone has ever suggested differently. In the innocent act of giving a place a pseudonym, we move from a world of specific occurrences, each happening for their own uniquely recurring reasons, to an ideal type of greater generality. There is something of trying to make the mundane grand in this: Yankee City rather than Newburyport, Massachusetts; Middletown rather than Muncie, Indiana. Pseudonyms are a rhetorical device to remind ethnographers of their native land that one does not use ethnography merely to produce a literal record of who said what to whom. Rather, one uses ethnography to produce a focused, analytic account about how some recurrent dilemma of social life is managed. Using pseudonyms, if it does nothing else, signals ethnographic intent, which is interpretive. Conversely, using real names signals an intent which is more committed to uncovering the single truth about X.

In this instance Nightingale Children's Center and its genetic counseling team have been created by me to describe how a set of workers with a service ideology which was committed to enlarging the autonomy of those who consult with them by using nondirective, value-neutral counseling techniques fared in one, admittedly not very representative pediatric hospital. My intent was to have the cases presented serve as springboards for thinking about a set of questions which vex me still, even as I try to write a last word about them.

This research occurred somewhere; exactly where is important, but beside the question. Some places I could have observed might have been much better at meeting user needs; others worse. However, none might have been so generous as Nightingale and its genetic counselors at providing so much diverse clinical material, so many of the problems that bedevil the definition, delivery, and evaluation of care and service.

The specific instances of care and service presented here all occurred a long time ago. There has been, as the previous chapter illustrates, much change in genetics and health care between the observation and the production of the text. Nonetheless, the core issues—the nature of and limits on lay and professional autonomy, the proper balance of individual and collective values in decision-making authority, the shadowy line between public and private domains—these have not changed, nor gotten easier to resolve, despite organizational innovations. This account points to some reasons why this might be so. By making someplace real into Nightingale, I intend to indicate just how general and widespread these difficulties are.

It seems to me that pseudonyms make ethnography possible in a context where the natives are likely to read and critique the analysis of their community, for the protection of anonymity allows subjects to participate in those small betrayals of one's intimates that make for such good data from the fieldworker's point of view. At the same time, the blurring of details at the margin, the changing of names and the like, provides subjects some deniability when a book makes its way back to the local arena on which it is based. In local communities, ethnographies of professional communities are read in the same spirit as any *roman à clef.* Ethnographers owe it to their subjects to make the decoding process as difficult as possible.

REFERENCES

Abbott, Andrew. 1981. "Status and Status Strain in the Professions." *American Journal of Sociology* 86:819–35.

Annas, George. 1983. "Baby Doe Regulations: Doctors as Child Abusers." *Hastings Center Report* 13:26–27.

———. 1991. "Ethics Committees: From Ethical Comfort to Ethical Cover." *Hastings Center Review* 21, no. 3:18–20.

Anspach, Renée R. 1988. "Notes on the Sociology of Medical Discourse: The Language of Case Presentation." *Journal of Health and Social Behavior* 29:357–75.

Antley, Ray. 1979. "The Genetic Counselor as Facilitator of the Counselee's Decision Process." In *Genetic Counseling: Facts, Values, and Norms* (Birth Defects: Original Article Series 15, no. 2), ed. Alexander Capron et al. New York: Allen R. Liss, 137–68.

Balin, Jane. 1988. "The Sacred Dimension of Pregnancy and Birth." *Qualitative Sociology* 11, no. 4:275–301.

Becker, Howard. 1970. *Sociological Work: Method and Substance*. Chicago: Aldine.

Becker, Howard, Blanche Geer, Everett C. Hughes, and Anselem Strauss. 1961. *Boys in White: Student Culture in Medical School*. Chicago: Univ. of Chicago Press.

Bittner, Egon. 1967a. "The Police on Skid Row." *American Sociological Review* 32:239–58.

Bittner, Egon. 1967b. "Police Discretion in the Apprehension of Mentally Ill Persons." *Social Problems* 14:278–92.

Bogdan, Robert, May Alice Brown, and Susan Bannerman Foster. 1982. "Be Honest But Not Cruel: Staff/Parent Communication on a Neonatal Unit." *Human Organization* 14:6–16.

Bosk, Charles L. 1979. *Forgive and Remember.* Chicago: Univ. of Chicago Press.

————. 1980. "Occupation Rituals in Patient Management." *New England Journal of Medicine* 303:71–76.

————. 1986. "The Social, Legal and Ethical Implications of Fetal Medicine." In *Genetics and Law,* vol. 3, ed. A. Milunsky and George Annas. New York: Plenum Press.

————. 1991. "Mistaking Identity: Medical Error, Plaintiff's Attorneys and Defendant Physicians." *Transactions & Studies of the College of Physicians of Philadelphia* 112, no. 3:249–61.

Bosk, Charles L., and Joel Frader. 1990. "AIDS and the Politics of the Shopfloor." *Milbank Memorial Fund Quarterly* 68, Supp. 2:257–79.

Broadhead, Robert. 1983. *The Private Lives and Professional Identity of Medical Students.* New Brunswick, NJ: Transaction Books.

Brown, Philip, and Edwin J. Mikkelson. 1990. *No Safe Place: Toxic Waste, Leukemia and Community Action.* Berkeley and Los Angeles: Univ. of California Press.

Bucher, R., and A. Strauss. 1961. "Professions in Process." *American Journal of Sociology* 66:325–34.

Burkett, Gary, and Kathleen Knafl. 1976. "Judgment and Decision-Making in a Medical Specialty." *Sociology of Work and Occupations* 1:82–109.

Canterbury v. Spence. 1972. 465 F.2d 772 (DC Cir.).

Chapoulle, Jean-Michel. 1987. "Everett C. Hughes and the Chicago School." *Urban Life* 15, nos. 3–4:259–98.

Clifford, James. 1988. *The Predicament of Culture: Twentieth-Century Ethnography, Literature and Art.* Cambridge, MA: Harvard Univ. Press.

Clifford, James, and George Marcus, eds. 1986. *Writing Culture: The Poetics and Politics of Ethnography.* Berkeley and Los Angeles: Univ. of California Press.

Coles, Robert. 1979. "Medical Ethics and Living a Life." *New England Journal of Medicine* 301, no. 8:444–46.

Coser, Lewis, 1974. *Greedy Institutions: Patterns of Undivided Commitment.* New York: Free Press.

Crane, D. 1976. *The Sanctity of Social Life: Physicians' Treatment of Critically Ill Patients.* Russel Sage Foundation, New York, 96–102.

Davis, Fred. 1959. "The Cab Driver and His Fare." *American Journal of Sociology* 65:158–65.

De Santis, Grace. 1980. "Realms of Expertise: A View from Within the Medical Profession." In *Research in The Sociology of Health Care.* Vol. 1. *Professional Control of Health Services and Challenges of Such Control.* Greenwich, CT: JAI Press, 179–236.

Douglas, M., and A. Wildavsky. 1982. *Risk and Culture: An Essay on the Selection of Technical and Environmental Dangers.* Berkeley: Univ. of California Press.

References

Drinnon, Richard. 1986. *Keeper of Concentration Camps: Dillon S. Meyer and American Concentration Camps*. Berkeley and Los Angeles: Univ. of California Press.

Duster, Troy. 1990. *Backdoor to Eugenics*. New York: Routledge.

Edgar, Harold, and David Rothman. 1990. "New Rules for New Drugs: The Challenge of AIDS to the Regulatory Process." *The Milbank Quarterly* 68, sup. 2: 111–42.

Epstein, Richard, Charles Gregory, and Harry Kolven, Jr. 1984. *Cases and Materials on Torts*. 4th ed. Boston: Little Brown.

Fletcher, J. C., and M. I. Evans. 1983. "Maternal Bonding in Early Fetal Ultrasound Examination." *New England Journal of Medicine* 308, no. 7 (February 17):392–93.

Fox, Renée C. 1959. *Experiment Perilous*. New York: Free Press.

Fox, Renée C., and Judith Swazey. 1974. *The Courage to Fail: A Social View of Organ Transplants and Dialysis*. Chicago: Univ. of Chicago Press, 109–49.

Frader, Joel, and Charles L. Bosk. 1981. "Parent Talk at Intensive Rounds." *Social Science and Medicine* 15E:267–74.

Fraser, Clark F. 1974. "Genetic Counseling." *American Journal of Human Genetics* 26:636–59.

Fraser, Clark F., and Abby Lippman-Hand. 1979. "Genetic Counseling— The Postcounseling Period: 1. Parents' Perceptions of Risk." *American Journal of Medical Genetics* 4:51–71.

Freidson, Eliot. 1970. *Professions in Medicine*. New York: Harper and Row.

———. 1976. *Doctoring Together*. New York: Elsevier.

Garfinkel, H. 1967. *Studies in Ethnomethodology*. Englewood Cliffs, NJ: Prentice-Hall.

Gerber, Lane. 1983. *Married to Their Careers: Career and Family Dilemmas in Doctors' Lives*. New York: Routledge.

Geertz, Clifford. 1976. "Thick Description." In *The Interpretation of Culture*. New York: Basic Books, 3–30.

Goffman, Erving. 1959. *The Presentation of Self in Everyday Life*. Garden City, NJ: Anchor Books.

———. 1961a. *Asylums: Essays on the Social Situation of Mental Patients and Other Inmates*. Garden City, NJ: Anchor Books, 85–152.

———. 1961b. *Stigma: Notes on the Management of Spoiled Identity*. Englewood Cliffs, NJ: Prentice-Hall.

———. 1961c. "Role Distance." In *Encounters*. Indianapolis and New York: Bobbs-Merrill, 85–152.

———. 1967. "Where the Action Is." In *Interactional Ritual*. New York: Pantheon, 149–270.

———. 1974. *Frame Analysis: An Essay on the Organization of Experience*. New York: Harper Books.

188

References

Gold, Ray. 1952. "Janitors versus Tenants: A Status Income Dilemma." *American Journal of Sociology* 57:486–93.

Goode, W. J. 1960. "Encroachment, Charlatanism, and the Emerging Profession: Psychology, Sociology, and Medicine." *American Sociological Review* 25:902–14.

Gould, Steven J. 1981. *The Mismeasure of Man.* New York: W. W. Norton.

Guillemin, Jean, and Eleanor Holmstrom. 1983. "Legal Cases, Government Regulations and Clinical Realities in Newborn Intensive Care." *American Journal of Perinatology* 1:89–97.

Guillemin, Jean, and Eleanor Holmstrom. 1986. *Mixed Blessings: Intensive Care for Newborns.* New York and Oxford: Oxford Univ. Press.

Gusfield, Joseph. 1981. *The Culture of Public Problems.* Chicago: Univ. of Chicago Press.

Haller, Mark H. 1963. *Eugenics: Hereditarian Attitudes in American Thought.* New Brunswick, NJ: Rutgers Univ. Press.

Hauerwaus, Stanley. 1977. "The Demands and Limits of Care: On the Moral Dilemmas of Neonatal Intensive Care." In *Truthfulness and Tragedy,* ed. Stanley Hauerwaus and R. Bondt. Notre Dame, IN: Univ. of Notre Dame Press.

Hilgartner, Steven. 1990. "The Dominant View of Popularization: Conceptual Problems, Political Issues." *Social Studies of Science* 20:519–39.

Hilgartner, Steven, and Charles L. Bosk. 1988. "The Rise and Fall of Social Problems: A Public Arenas Model." *American Journal of Sociology* 94:53–78.

Hochschild, Arlie Russell. 1983. *The Managed Heart: Commercialization of Human Feeling.* Berkeley and Los Angeles: Univ. of California Press.

Hoffmaster, Barry. 1990. "Can Ethnography Save the Life of Medical Ethics?" (mimeo).

Hughes, Everett, C. 1971. *The Sociological Eye: Selected Papers on Work, Self, and Society.* Chicago: Aldine-Atherton.

Hunter, Kathryn. 1991. *Doctors' Stories: The Narrative Structure of Medical Knowledge.* Princeton, NJ: Princeton Univ. Press.

Imber, Jonathan. B. 1986. *Abortion and the Private Practice of Medicine.* New Haven, CT: Yale Univ. Press.

Jacobs, Mark. 1990. *Screwing the System and Making It Work.* Chicago: Univ. of Chicago Press.

Joffe, Carol. 1987. *The Regulation of Sexuality.* Philadelphia: Temple Univ. Press.

Jones, James H. 1981. *Bad Blood: The Tuskegee Syphilis Experiment.* New York: Free Press.

Kass, Leon. 1972. "Making Babies: The New Biology and the 'Old' Morality." *Public Interest* 26:18–56.

Kessler, Seymour. 1980. "The Psychological Paradigm Shift in Genetic Counseling." *Social Biology* 27:167–85.

Kaback, Michael. 1977. "Tay-Sachs Disease: From Clinical Description to Prospective Control." In *Tay-Sachs Disease: Screening and Prevention* (Birth Defects: Original Articles Series), ed. D. Bergsma and Michael Kaback. New York: Allan Liss.

Kolata. 1990. *The Baby-Doctors: Probing the Limits of Fetal Medicine.* New York: Delacorte.

Lévi-Strauss, Claude. 1966. *The Savage Mind.* Chicago: Univ. of Chicago Press.

Lidz, C., A. Meisel, E. Zerubavel, M. Caster, R. Sestak, and L. Roth. 1984. *Informed Consent: A Study of Decision Making in Psychiatry.* New York: Guilford Press.

Lifton, Robert J. 1986. *The Nazi Doctors.* New York: Basic Books.

Light, David, L. 1980. *Becoming Psychiatrists: The Professional Transformation of Self.* New York: W. W. Norton.

Light, Donald. 1972. "Psychiatry and Suicide: The Management of a Mistake." *American Journal of Sociology* 77:821–38.

Lippman-Hand, Abby, and Clark F. Fraser. 1979. "Genetic Counseling—The Postcounseling Period: Parents' Perceptions of Uncertainty." *American Journal of Medical Genetics* 4:51–71.

Lowe, C., D. Alexander, D. Bryla, and D. Seigel. 1978. *The Safety and Accuracy of Mid-Trimester Amniocentesis.* DHEW Pub. No. (N114), 78–190.

Ludmerer, Kenneth. 1972. *Genetics and American Society.* Baltimore: Johns Hopkins Univ. Press.

Lukas, Antony. 1991. "The Fire This Time." *American Prospect* 5:102–14.

Luker, Kristin. 1984. *Abortion and the Politics of Motherhood.* Berkeley and Los Angeles: Univ. of California Press.

Marks, Joan. 1991. "The Training of Genetic Counselors: Origins of a Psychosocial Model." Paper presented at a workshop: Genetic Counseling: Ethics, Values, Professional Responsibilities. Univ. of Minnesota.

Matza, David. 1964. *Delinquency and Drift.* New York: John Wiley.

Merton, Robert K. 1973. *The Sociology of Science: Theoretical and Empirical Investigations.* Chicago: Univ. of Chicago Press, 267–78.

———. 1968. *Social Theory and Social Structure.* New York: Free Press, 441–74.

Miller, Steven J. 1970. *Prescription for Leadership: Training for the Medical Elite.* Chicago: Aldine.

Millman, Marcia. 1976. *The Unkindest Cut: Life in the Backrooms of Medicine.* New York: William Morrow.

Murray, T. 1985. "The Final Anticlimatic Ruling on Baby Doe." *Hastings Center Report* 15:5–9.

Nisbet, Robert. 1976. *Sociology as an Art Form.* New York: Oxford University Press.

Olshansky, Simon. 1973. "Chronic Sorrow: A Response to Having a Mentally Defective Child." *Social Casework* 10:129–34.

Parsons, Talcott. 1951. *The Social System.* Glencoe, IL: Free Press, 428–79.

Perrow, Charles. 1985. *Normal Accidents: Living with High-Risk Technologies.* New York: Basic Books.

Proctor, Robert. 1988. *Racial Hygiene: Medicine Under the Nazi.* Cambridge, MA: Harvard Univ. Press.

Rabinow, Paul. 1977. *Reflections on Fieldwork in Morocco.* Berkeley and Los Angeles: Univ. of California Press.

Rabinow, Paul, and William Sullivan. 1979. *Interpretive Social Science.* Berkeley and Los Angeles: Univ. of California Press.

Rhoden, D., and G. Annas. 1985. "Withholding Treatment from Baby Doe." *Milbank Quarterly* 63:18–51.

Reed, Sheldon. 1974. "A Short History of Human Genetics in the USA." *Social Biology* 21:332–39.

Reilly, Philip. 1987. "Involuntary Sterilization in the United States: A Surgical Solution." *Quarterly Review of Biology* 67:153–70.

Robertson, J. 1981. "Dilemma in Danville." *Hastings Center Report* 11, no. 5:5–8.

Roe v. Wade. 1973. 410 U.S. 116.

Rosenberg, Charles. 1974. "Hereditary Disease and Social Thought." *Perspectives in American History* 8:189–235.

———. 1976. "The Bitter Fault: Heredity, Disease and Social Thought." In *No Other Gods: On Science and Social Thought.* Baltimore: Johns Hopkins Univ. Press, 25–53.

———. 1987. *The Care of Strangers: The Rise of America's Hospital System.* New York: Basic Books.

Rosenstock, Irwin, B. Childs, and A. M. Simopoulous. 1975. *Genetic Screening.* Washington, DC: National Academy of Science.

Rothman, David. 1991. *Strangers at Bedside: How Law and Bioethics Transformed American Medicine.* New York: Basic Books.

Roy, Donald. 1952. "Quota Restriction and Goldbricking in a Machine Shop." *American Journal of Sociology* 57:427–42.

Scheff, Thomas, J. 1968. "Negotiating Reality: Notes on Power in the Assessment of Responsibility." *Social Problems* 16:3–17.

Schneider, J. 1985. "The Social Construction of Social Problems." *Annual Review of Sociology* 11:209–29.

Schutz, Alfred. 1971. *Collected Papers 1: The Problem of Social Reality.* The Hague: Martinus Nyhoff, 207–59.

Scully, Diana. 1980. *Men Who Control Women's Health: The Miseducation of Obstetrician-Gynecologists.* Boston: Houghton Mifflin.

Shem, Samuel. 1978. *The House of God.* New York: Richard Marek.

Siegler, Mark. 1975. "Pascal's Wager and the Hanging of Crepe." *New England Journal of Medicine* 293:853–57.

Silverman, William. 1981. "Mismatched Attitudes about Neonatal Death." *Hastings Center Report* 11:12–17.

Sorenson, J., and A. Cuthbert. 1979. "Professional Orientations to Contemporary Genetic Counseling." In *Genetic Counseling: Facts, Values, and Norms* (Birth Defects: Original Article Series, 15, no. 2), ed. Alexander Capron et al. New York: Allen R. Liss, 85–102.

Stelling, Joan, and Rue Bucher. 1972. "Autonomy and Monitoring in Hospital Wards." *Sociological Quarterly* 13:431–47.

Stinson, Robert, and Peggy Stinson. 1979. "On the Death of a Baby." *Atlantic Monthly* 1979:64–72.

———. 1983. *The Long Dying of Baby Andrew.* Boston and Toronto: Atlantic Monthly Press Book—Little Brown, 1983.

Strauss, Anselm, S. Fazerhaugh, B. Suczek, and C. Wiener. 1985. *The Social Organization of Medical Work.* Chicago: Univ. of Chicago Press.

Strauss, Anselm, F. Schatzman, F. R. Becher et al. 1964. *Psychiatric Ideologies and Institutions.* Glencoe, IL: Free Press.

Sudnow, David. 1967. *Passing On: The Social Organization of Dying.* Englewood Cliffs, NJ: Prentice-Hall.

Suzuki, David, and Peter Knudtson. 1990. *Genethics: The Ethics of Engineering Life.* Cambridge, MA: Harvard Univ. Press.

Tancredi, Lawrence, J., and Dorothy Nelkin. 1989. *Dangerous Diagnostics: The Social Power of Biological Information.* New York: Basic Books.

Twiss, Sumner B. 1979. "The Genetic Counselor as Moral Advisor." In *Genetic Counseling: Facts, Values, and Norms.* (Birth Defects: Original Articles Series, 15, no. 2), ed. Alexander Capron et al. New York: Alan R. Liss, 201–12.

Van Maanen, John. 1988. *Tales from the Field.* 1988. Chicago: Univ. of Chicago Press.

Weber, Max. 1958. *The Protestant Ethic and The Spirit of Capitalism.* New York: Charles Scribner's Sons.

Webster v. Missouri Reproductive Services. 1989. 492 U.S. 490.

Wertz, Dorothy, and John Fletcher. 1988. "Attitudes of Genetic Counselors: A Multinational Survey." *American Journal of Human Genetics* 42:592–600.

Wertz, Dorothy, and John Fletcher, eds. 1989. *Ethics and Genetics: A Cross-Cultural Perspective.* New York: Springer-Verlag.

Wertz, Dorothy, John Fletcher, and John Mulvihill. 1990. "Medical Geneticists Confront Ethical Dilemmas: Cross-Cultural Comparisons Among 18 Nations." *American Journal of Human Genetics* 46:1200–1213.

Yarborough, M., J. A. Scott, and L. K. Dixon. 1989. "The Role of Beneficence in Clinical Genetics: Non-Directive Counseling Reconsidered. *Theoretical Medicine* 10(2):139–49.

Zerubavel, Eviatar. 1979. *Patterns of Time in Hospital Life: A Sociological Perspective.* Chicago: Univ. of Chicago Press.

Zussman, Robert. 1992. *Intensive Care.* Chicago: Univ. of Chicago Press.

INDEX